KATE HALE

Pregnancy Myths and Facts

Separating Truth from Misconceptions

Contents

Introduction

Pregnancy is one of the most trans-formative and life-changing experiences a woman can go through. It's a time filled with excitement, anticipation, and often, uncertainty. For centuries, people have passed down stories, advice, and beliefs about pregnancy—some rooted in cultural traditions, others in personal anecdotes. While many of these ideas can be well-intentioned, they can also be misleading. In today's world, the abundance of information from social media, family, friends, and even outdated medical advice can leave many women confused about what is true and what is myth. Understanding these myths and their impact on pregnant women is essential to navigating this special time in a woman's life.

Many pregnancy myths have persisted for generations, passed from one person to another, until they become ingrained in the collective understanding of pregnancy. These myths can range from harmless misconceptions, like believing the baby's gender can be determined by the shape of the mother's belly, to potentially harmful ones, like avoiding vaccinations or certain foods. The spread of misinformation can leave women feeling anxious, stressed, and unsure of what choices to make. Myths can influence everything from nutrition and exercise to labor and delivery decisions, often leading women to make choices that are not based on science or medical advice. In fact, the overwhelming nature of conflicting information can create unnecessary fear and anxiety during what should be an exciting and joyful time.

One of the biggest challenges for expecting mothers today is determining which information is accurate. The internet, while a great resource, is also a major contributor to the spread of pregnancy myths. Blogs, forums, and social media platforms are filled with opinions and experiences that may or may not be based on evidence. It's not uncommon for expectant mothers to be inundated with advice from well-meaning friends and family members, who often share outdated or incorrect beliefs about pregnancy. This can create confusion, especially when myths contradict medical advice provided by healthcare professionals.

The prevalence of these myths can have real consequences. For example, misconceptions about nutrition and exercise can lead women to make unhealthy choices during pregnancy. Misinformation about labor and delivery can cause fear and anxiety about the birthing process. Myths about breastfeeding and postpartum recovery can leave new mothers feeling overwhelmed and unprepared for the realities of caring for a newborn. In some cases, these myths can even lead to dangerous decisions, such as avoiding necessary medical interventions or treatments. It's crucial for women to be able to separate fact from fiction, especially during pregnancy when their health and the health of their baby are at stake.

This book was written to address these myths head-on, providing expecting mothers with accurate, evidence-based information that they can rely on. By separating fact from fiction, this book aims to empower women to make informed decisions throughout their pregnancy journey. The goal is to provide clarity and confidence, helping women feel more in control during this trans-formative time. Whether it's understanding the truth behind common gender prediction myths or learning about the importance of proper nutrition and exercise during pregnancy, this book covers a wide range of topics that are relevant to expecting mothers.

Why is this book important? Because misinformation about pregnancy is not just frustrating—it can be harmful. The decisions women make during pregnancy can have lasting effects on their health and the health of their baby. Having access to accurate information is essential for making informed choices, whether it's about prenatal care, labor and delivery, or postpartum recovery. This book provides a comprehensive guide to debunking common pregnancy myths and offering factual, science-backed information that women can trust.

Pregnancy myths often stem from cultural traditions, anecdotal experiences, or outdated medical practices. While some myths may seem harmless, they can lead to confusion and, in some cases, dangerous decisions. For example, the myth that pregnant women should avoid exercise can prevent women from engaging in physical activity that could benefit both their health and their baby's development. Similarly, the myth that certain foods should be avoided during pregnancy may lead to unnecessary dietary restrictions, depriving women of important nutrients. By providing accurate information, this book helps women make decisions that are in their best interest and that of their baby.

Throughout this book, you will find clear explanations of common pregnancy myths, along with the facts that dispel them. Each chapter is designed to tackle a specific area of pregnancy, from nutrition and exercise to labor and delivery. The information is based on current medical research and expert advice, ensuring that readers can trust the guidance they are receiving. By the end of this book, you will have a better understanding of what is true and what is false when it comes to pregnancy, allowing you to make informed choices and feel confident in your decisions.

One of the key features of this book is its practical approach. While it is important to understand the facts behind pregnancy myths, it is equally important to know how to apply that knowledge in real life. This book provides practical tips and advice that expecting mothers can use throughout their pregnancy. Whether it's creating a balanced meal plan, developing a safe exercise routine, or preparing for labor, this book offers actionable steps that can help women have a healthy and positive pregnancy experience. The goal is not just to provide information, but to help women feel empowered and confident in their ability to make the best choices for themselves and their baby.

So, how should you use this book? Consider it a guide that you can refer to throughout your pregnancy. Each chapter is designed to address a specific area of concern, making it easy to find the information you need when you need it. If you're unsure about a particular myth or piece of advice you've heard, you can flip to the relevant chapter to find out whether it's true or false. This book is also a great resource to share with your partner, family members, or friends, helping them understand the facts about pregnancy and dispelling any misconceptions they may have.

One of the biggest challenges in navigating pregnancy is dealing with the sheer amount of information available. From doctors and midwives to friends, family, and the internet, there's no shortage of advice when it comes to pregnancy. But not all advice is created equal, and it can be difficult to know which sources to trust. This book aims to cut through the noise, providing expecting mothers with the information they need to make informed decisions. By understanding the facts behind pregnancy myths, women can feel more confident in their choices and less overwhelmed by conflicting advice.

Pregnancy is a time of great change, both physically and emotionally. It's a time when women need support, understanding, and accurate information. This book was written to provide that support, offering women a reliable resource that they can turn to throughout their pregnancy. Whether you're a first-time mom or an experienced parent, this book offers valuable insights that can help you navigate the challenges and joys of pregnancy. By debunking common myths and providing factual information, this book empowers women to make informed decisions and have a healthy, positive pregnancy experience.

INTRODUCTION

The journey to understanding pregnancy is not always straightforward. There are countless myths and misconceptions that can make it difficult to know what's true and what's not. But by educating yourself and seeking out reliable information, you can feel more confident in your decisions and better prepared for the challenges of pregnancy. This book is designed to help you do just that—separate fact from fiction and make informed choices that are in the best interest of you and your baby.

As you read through the chapters of this book, you will gain a deeper understanding of the common myths and misconceptions surrounding pregnancy. Each chapter is packed with evidence-based information, providing you with the tools you need to make informed decisions. Whether it's understanding the truth about exercise during pregnancy, learning about the realities of labor and delivery, or debunking myths about postpartum recovery, this book offers a comprehensive guide to navigating pregnancy with confidence.

Pregnancy is a time of joy and anticipation, but it can also be a time of uncertainty. The goal of this book is to provide clarity and support, helping women feel more informed and empowered as they navigate this special time in their lives. By separating fact from fiction, this book aims to reduce the anxiety and confusion that often comes with pregnancy myths. Instead, it offers a clear path forward, providing women with the knowledge they need to make the best choices for themselves and their baby.

At the heart of this book is the belief that every woman deserves to have a positive and healthy pregnancy experience. By debunking common myths and providing accurate information, this book empowers women to take control of their pregnancy journey. Whether you're just starting out or are well into your pregnancy, this book offers valuable insights that can help you feel more confident and informed. It's time to put an end to the confusion and misinformation and embrace the truth about pregnancy.

The journey to understanding pregnancy begins with knowledge. By educating yourself about the facts and dispelling the myths, you can take control of your pregnancy and feel more confident in your decisions. This book is your guide to navigating the world of pregnancy myths and misconceptions, offering clear, evidence-based information that you can rely on. Whether you're a first-time mom or an experienced parent, this book will help you separate fact from fiction and make informed choices throughout your pregnancy journey.

Common Early Pregnancy Myths

Pregnancy is a time filled with anticipation, joy, and sometimes confusion. One of the main sources of uncertainty for many women is the sheer number of myths that surround early pregnancy. These myths often stem from outdated beliefs, cultural traditions, or anecdotal stories passed down through generations. While some myths may seem harmless, others can lead to misconceptions that impact decision-making during this crucial time. In this chapter, we will address three common early pregnancy myths, break them down, and present the scientific facts that separate truth from fiction.

Myth 1: You Can't Get Pregnant While Breastfeeding

One of the most widespread myths about early pregnancy is the belief that breastfeeding serves as a natural contraceptive. Many new mothers are told that as long as they are breastfeeding, they cannot get pregnant. This myth is often based on the natural hormonal changes that occur during breastfeeding, which can delay ovulation. However, while breastfeeding can impact fertility, it is by no means a foolproof method of birth control.

To understand why this myth persists, it's essential to look at how breastfeeding affects a woman's body. During breastfeeding, the hormone prolactin, which is responsible for milk production, also suppresses ovulation. This process is known as lactational amenorrhea, and in some women, it can delay the return of menstruation and ovulation for several months. As a result, some women do not ovulate or have periods while they are exclusively breastfeeding, particularly in the first six months postpartum. This phenomenon can give the impression that breastfeeding prevents pregnancy.

However, lactational amenorrhea is only effective as a method of birth control under specific conditions. According to the World Health Organization (WHO), breastfeeding can act as a contraceptive method, but only when:
- The baby is less than six months old.
- The mother is exclusively breastfeeding, meaning the baby is not receiving any supplemental food or formula.
- The mother's menstrual cycle has not yet returned.

Once any of these conditions change—such as the introduction of solid foods, decreased breastfeeding frequency, or the return of menstruation—ovulation can resume. It's important to note that ovulation can occur before the first postpartum period, meaning that a woman can become fertile without realizing it. This is why many women are surprised when they find out they are pregnant despite breastfeeding.

For women who wish to avoid pregnancy during the breastfeeding period, relying solely on breastfeeding as a form of birth control is not recommended. It is essential to use additional contraceptive methods if pregnancy prevention is the goal. Barrier methods such as condoms, as well as non-hormonal or progestin-only birth control options, are considered safe for breastfeeding mothers. Women should consult with their healthcare provider to discuss the best contraceptive options for their individual circumstances.

In conclusion, while breastfeeding can temporarily suppress fertility in some women, it is not a reliable long-term method of contraception. The return of ovulation can be unpredictable, and relying on breastfeeding alone to prevent pregnancy carries a significant risk of unintended conception.

Myth 2: Morning Sickness Only Happens in the Morning

Morning sickness is one of the most common symptoms of early pregnancy, and for many women, it can be one of the first signs that they are expecting. However, despite its name, the idea that morning sickness only occurs in the morning is a myth. The reality is that nausea and vomiting can happen at any time of day or night during pregnancy.

The term "morning sickness" likely originated because, for some women, nausea can feel more pronounced in the morning when the stomach is empty. However, hormonal fluctuations during pregnancy, particularly the increase in human chorionic gonadotropin (hCG) and estrogen, are responsible for triggering nausea, and these hormones do not operate on a strict morning schedule. For this reason, many women experience nausea throughout the day, or even exclusively in the afternoon or evening.

Research shows that up to 70-80% of pregnant women experience nausea and vomiting during the first trimester. For most women, these symptoms typically begin around the sixth week of pregnancy and start to subside by the end of the first trimester, although for some, they can persist longer. The severity and timing of morning sickness can vary widely from one woman to another. Some women may only feel mildly queasy, while others may experience severe nausea and vomiting throughout the day, a condition known as hypertensives gravidarum.

There are several factors that may contribute to why some women experience nausea at different times of the day. Low blood sugar levels, fatigue, and an empty stomach can all exacerbate nausea, which is why some women feel worse in the morning after a night of fasting. However, the rising and falling levels of pregnancy hormones like hCG and estrogen, as well as heightened sensitivity to certain smells and tastes, can trigger nausea at any point during the day. For example, exposure to strong odors or certain foods can bring on a wave of nausea, regardless of the time.

It is also important to recognize that morning sickness is a natural part of pregnancy and is generally considered a sign of a healthy pregnancy. In fact, studies have shown that women who experience nausea and vomiting in early pregnancy have a lower risk of miscarriage, although this does not mean that the absence of morning sickness indicates a problem.

To manage morning sickness, women can try a variety of strategies to reduce nausea, such as eating small, frequent meals, avoiding foods that trigger nausea, staying hydrated, and getting plenty of rest. Some women find relief from natural remedies such as ginger, peppermint, or acupressure wristbands. In more severe cases, healthcare providers may prescribe anti-nausea medications that are safe for pregnancy.

In conclusion, morning sickness is a misnomer because nausea and vomiting during pregnancy can occur at any time of day or night. While the symptoms can be unpleasant, they are a normal part of pregnancy for many women. By understanding the underlying causes and adopting strategies to manage symptoms, women can find relief and reassurance that morning sickness is typically a temporary phase of early pregnancy.

Myth 3: Stress Can Prevent You from Getting Pregnant

The idea that stress can prevent pregnancy is another common myth that many women encounter when trying to conceive. While stress can certainly have an impact on overall health and well-being, the notion that stress alone can prevent pregnancy is not entirely accurate. Fertility is influenced by a wide range of factors, including age, hormonal balance, reproductive health, and lifestyle choices. Stress, while it can affect the body in various ways, is unlikely to be the sole cause of infertility.

Stress is a natural response to challenging situations, and it triggers the release of hormones such as cortisol and adrenaline. Chronic stress, however, can disrupt the body's hormonal balance, which may affect reproductive health to some extent. For example, in extreme cases of chronic stress, women may experience disruptions in their menstrual cycle, such as irregular periods or amenorrhea (the absence of menstruation). This is because high levels of stress hormones can interfere with the production of reproductive hormones like estrogen and progesterone, which regulate ovulation and menstruation.

That being said, the idea that stress alone can prevent pregnancy is an oversimplification. Most women who experience stress will continue to ovulate and have regular menstrual cycles, and many women who are under stress can and do conceive. It's important to recognize that fertility is a complex process that involves many physiological factors, and while stress may play a role, it is rarely the sole determining factor.

In fact, studies on the relationship between stress and fertility have produced mixed results. Some research suggests that high levels of stress may slightly reduce the chances of conception, but other studies have found no significant correlation between stress and infertility. It is likely that the effects of stress on fertility vary from woman to woman, and other factors such as age, underlying health conditions, and lifestyle habits (such as smoking or alcohol use) may play a more significant role in determining fertility.

It is also important to acknowledge the emotional toll that infertility can take on couples trying to conceive. The pressure to become pregnant can itself become a source of stress, leading to a vicious cycle where the stress of trying to conceive adds to the emotional burden. In such cases, it can be helpful for couples to seek support from healthcare providers, counselors, or support groups to address the emotional aspects of fertility challenges.

While reducing stress is generally beneficial for overall health, it is not a guaranteed solution to fertility issues. Women who are concerned about their fertility should seek advice from a healthcare provider to assess potential underlying causes of infertility, such as hormonal imbalances, reproductive health conditions (e.g., polycystic ovary syndrome or endometriosis), or age-related fertility decline.

In conclusion, while chronic stress may have some impact on reproductive health, it is not a definitive cause of infertility. Stress is just one of many factors that can influence fertility, and women who are trying to conceive should focus on maintaining a healthy lifestyle, managing stress, and seeking medical advice if they encounter difficulties in becoming pregnant.

Scientific Facts Behind Early Pregnancy Changes

Early pregnancy is a time of profound physiological changes, many of which are triggered by hormonal shifts that support the growth and development of the embryo. Understanding these changes can help dispel myths and provide clarity about what to expect in the early stages of pregnancy.

One of the first and most important changes that occur in early pregnancy is the rise in human chorionic gonadotropin (hCG) levels. This hormone, produced by the placenta, is responsible for maintaining the corpus luteum, which in turn produces progesterone to support the pregnancy. hCG is also the hormone detected by pregnancy tests, and its levels rise rapidly in the first few weeks of pregnancy. High hCG levels are associated with many of the early symptoms of pregnancy, including nausea and vomiting (morning sickness).

Progesterone and estrogen levels also increase during early pregnancy, playing critical roles in preparing the body for pregnancy. Progesterone helps maintain the uterine lining and prevents contractions, while estrogen supports the development of the placenta and feàtal organs. These hormonal changes can cause a variety of physical and emotional symptoms, such as fatigue, mood swings, breast tenderness, and food aversions or cravings. While these symptoms can be uncomfortable, they are normal and typically subside as the pregnancy progresses.

Another significant change during early pregnancy is the increased blood flow to support the growing fetus. The body begins to produce more blood, leading to changes in circulation and sometimes causing symptoms like dizziness or lightheadedness. The cardiovascular system adapts to the increased demand by enlarging the blood vessels and slightly lowering blood pressure. This adjustment helps ensure that both the mother and the fetus receive adequate oxygen and nutrients.

The digestive system also undergoes changes in early pregnancy. Progesterone, which relaxes smooth muscles, slows down the digestive process, which can lead to common pregnancy symptoms such as bloating, constipation, and heartburn. These symptoms are a result of the digestive tract becoming less efficient in moving food through the intestines, allowing more time for nutrients to be absorbed and directed to the developing baby. While this slowdown can be uncomfortable, it is a normal part of pregnancy and can often be managed with dietary changes and lifestyle adjustments.

In addition to physical changes, early pregnancy is also marked by emotional and psychological adjustments. Hormonal fluctuations can contribute to mood swings, anxiety, and changes in emotional responses. Many women experience heightened emotions, ranging from joy and excitement to worry and stress about the health of the baby and the changes in their own bodies. It's important to recognize that these emotional shifts are normal and that seeking support from partners, healthcare providers, or mental health professionals can be beneficial in managing the emotional challenges of pregnancy.

One of the most commonly misunderstood aspects of early pregnancy is the timing of ovulation and conception. Many women believe that conception occurs immediately after intercourse, but in reality, sperm can live inside the female reproductive tract for up to five days, waiting for an egg to be released. Ovulation typically occurs about 14 days before the start of the next menstrual period, but the exact timing can vary depending on the length of a woman's menstrual cycle. Conception occurs when a sperm fertilizes an egg, and the fertilized egg then travels to the uterus, where it implants in the uterine lining. This process can take several days, which is why women may not experience pregnancy symptoms right away.

It's also important to note that not all women experience the same symptoms during early pregnancy. Some women may have noticeable symptoms, such as nausea, breast tenderness, and fatigue, within a few weeks of conception, while others may not experience any symptoms until later in the first trimester. Every pregnancy is unique, and the intensity and timing of symptoms can vary widely.

In terms of early pregnancy health, one of the most crucial factors is prenatal care. Women should seek medical advice as soon as they suspect they are pregnant to confirm the pregnancy and ensure they receive appropriate care. Prenatal care includes regular checkups, ultrasounds, and tests to monitor the health of both the mother and the baby. During these visits, healthcare providers can offer guidance on nutrition, exercise, and managing pregnancy symptoms, as well as screen for any potential complications.

One of the most effective ways to debunk pregnancy myths is through education and access to accurate, evidence-based information. Understanding the scientific facts behind early pregnancy changes can help women make informed decisions about their health and well-being. For example, while it's common to hear that certain foods or activities should be avoided during pregnancy, it's important to consult with a healthcare provider to get accurate advice tailored to individual needs. Similarly, staying informed about the normal symptoms and changes of early pregnancy can help alleviate unnecessary worry and anxiety.

In summary, early pregnancy is a time of significant physical, hormonal, and emotional changes. While many myths persist about what is normal or expected during this time, the scientific facts paint a clearer picture of what happens inside the body during the first trimester. Understanding these changes can help women feel more prepared and confident as they navigate their pregnancy journey. Whether it's learning the truth behind common misconceptions or gaining a better understanding of the hormonal and physiological processes that support pregnancy, knowledge is a powerful tool in ensuring a healthy and positive experience.

The importance of debunking myths and spreading factual information cannot be overstated. Misinformation can lead to unnecessary stress and confusion, which may impact a woman's ability to enjoy her pregnancy fully. By separating myths from facts, women can focus on what truly matters— taking care of their health and the health of their growing baby. Whether it's addressing misconceptions about fertility, morning sickness, or the effects of stress, this chapter serves as a guide to helping women navigate the early stages of pregnancy with clarity and confidence.

Ultimately, every woman's pregnancy experience is unique, and while certain symptoms and changes are common, each journey is different. By relying on accurate information and staying in close contact with healthcare professionals, women can feel empowered to make informed choices that support their well-being. As we continue through the book, the aim is to provide clear, evidence-based guidance that debunks myths and offers practical advice for a healthy, joyful pregnancy.

Gender Predictions

The excitement and curiosity surrounding a baby's gender have long fascinated expectant parents, often leading to a slew of gender prediction methods. While some people wait until the baby's birth to discover their gender, many others eagerly anticipate finding out as early as possible. Modern science offers accurate methods to determine a baby's gender, but throughout history and across cultures, numerous gender prediction myths and old wives' tales have persisted. These myths often involve observations of physical changes, behaviors, or cravings during pregnancy, which supposedly reveal whether the baby is a boy or a girl. In this chapter, we will delve into some of the most common gender prediction myths, including the shape of the belly, heart rate, and food cravings, and examine the scientific evidence behind these beliefs.

Myth 4: The Shape of Your Belly Can Predict the Baby's Gender

One of the most well-known and enduring gender prediction myths is that the shape of a pregnant woman's belly can reveal the sex of her baby. According to this belief, if a woman is carrying her baby high and her belly is round, she is likely having a girl. Conversely, if her belly is low and more pointed, she is said to be carrying a boy. This myth is often shared by well-meaning friends, family members, and even strangers, who believe they can accurately predict the baby's gender simply by looking at the shape of the mother's abdomen.

The origin of this myth is unclear, but it has been passed down through generations in many different cultures. The idea behind the myth is that the baby's gender influences how the mother carries the baby, with boys supposedly being carried lower and girls being carried higher. However, there is no scientific basis for this belief, and numerous studies have debunked the idea that the shape or position of the belly can predict the baby's gender.

The shape of a pregnant woman's belly is determined by several factors, none of which are related to the baby's gender. One of the primary factors is the position of the baby in the uterus. As the baby grows and moves, their position can change, which in turn affects how the belly appears from the outside. Additionally, the mother's body type, the tone of her abdominal muscles, and whether she has been pregnant before all play a role in determining the shape and position of her belly.

For example, women who have strong abdominal muscles may carry their baby higher, while those with weaker abdominal muscles, especially women who have had multiple pregnancies, may carry lower. The amount of amniotic fluid surrounding the baby can also influence the size and shape of the belly. Furthermore, as the pregnancy progresses and the baby grows, the shape of the belly may change, making it difficult to use belly shape as a reliable indicator of the baby's gender.

Medical professionals, including obstetricians and midwives, emphasize that the shape of the belly has no bearing on the sex of the baby. Ultrasounds and other medical procedures, such as non-invasive prenatal testing (NIPT) or amniocentesis, are the only reliable ways to determine the baby's gender before birth. These methods provide accurate information by examining the baby's chromosomes or anatomy, not the mother's physical appearance.

Despite the lack of scientific evidence supporting the belly shape myth, it continues to be a popular topic of conversation among pregnant women and their social circles. For many, guessing the baby's gender based on the shape of the belly is seen as a harmless and fun activity. However, it's important for expectant parents to understand that this method is not based on fact and should not be relied upon for making any decisions or assumptions about the baby's gender.

Myth 5: Heart Rate Predicts the Baby's Gender

Another common myth about gender prediction is the belief that the baby's heart rate can reveal whether the baby is a boy or a girl. According to this myth, if the baby's heart rate is above 140 beats per minute (bpm), the baby is likely a girl. If the heart rate is below 140 bpm, the baby is supposedly a boy. This idea is often shared during prenatal visits when the baby's heart rate is measured using a Doppler device or during an ultrasound.

The origin of this myth may be rooted in the general observation that female and male adults have different average heart rates, with women typically having slightly faster heart rates than men. However, applying this concept to a developing fetus is not scientifically accurate. The baby's heart rate is influenced by a variety of factors, including gestational age, activity level, and overall health, none of which are related to the baby's gender.

In the early stages of pregnancy, the baby's heart rate is generally much faster than that of an adult. During the first trimester, it is not uncommon for the fetal heart rate to be between 120 and 160 bpm, regardless of the baby's gender. As the pregnancy progresses, the heart rate may fluctuate based on the baby's activity level and growth, but there is no consistent difference between the heart rates of male and female fetuses.

Several scientific studies have examined the relationship between fetal heart rate and gender, and the results consistently show that there is no significant correlation. One such study, published in the journal *Fetal Diagnosis and Therapy*, analyzed the heart rates of over 500 fetuses during early pregnancy and found no consistent pattern that could be used to predict the baby's gender. The study concluded that heart rate is not a reliable indicator of gender and that other factors, such as the baby's movements or the mother's physical condition, are more likely to influence heart rate fluctuations.

It is also important to note that heart rate can vary throughout the day and may change in response to factors such as the baby's activity level, maternal stress, or even the time of day. A higher heart rate during one prenatal visit does not necessarily mean that the baby's heart rate will remain high throughout the pregnancy, nor does it provide any insight into the baby's gender.

Like the belly shape myth, the heart rate myth is often treated as a fun guessing game among friends and family members. However, it is not based on scientific evidence, and expectant parents should not rely on heart rate measurements to determine the sex of their baby. Accurate gender determination can only be achieved through medical tests, such as an ultrasound or genetic testing.

Myth 6: Cravings Reveal Gender

One of the more entertaining and widely believed gender prediction myths is the idea that a pregnant woman's food cravings can reveal the gender of her baby. According to this myth, women who crave sweet foods, such as chocolate, fruit, or desserts, are likely carrying a girl. On the other hand, women who crave salty or savory foods, such as chips, pickles, or meat, are supposedly carrying a boy. This belief is often shared in casual conversations, and many women enjoy comparing their cravings with the predicted gender of their baby.

The concept of cravings as a gender predictor is intriguing, but there is no scientific basis for this myth. Food cravings during pregnancy are common, and they can vary widely from woman to woman and even from pregnancy to pregnancy. Cravings are influenced by a range of factors, including hormonal changes, nutritional needs, cultural influences, and even emotional factors, but there is no evidence to suggest that they are linked to the baby's gender.

Pregnancy hormones, particularly estrogen and progesterone, play a significant role in influencing taste and smell, which may explain why some women develop strong cravings for certain foods during pregnancy. Additionally, changes in blood sugar levels or nutritional deficiencies can trigger cravings for specific nutrients, such as carbohydrates, proteins, or fats. For example, a woman who is low in iron may crave red meat, while a woman with low blood sugar may crave sugary snacks. These cravings are the body's way of signaling a need for specific nutrients, rather than an indicator of the baby's gender.

Cultural and psychological factors can also influence pregnancy cravings. In some cultures, certain foods are believed to be beneficial or harmful during pregnancy, which may lead women to crave or avoid those foods based on cultural beliefs. Emotional factors, such as stress or comfort-seeking behavior, can also contribute to cravings. For example, a woman who is feeling anxious or overwhelmed may crave familiar comfort foods, such as sweets or salty snacks, as a way to soothe her emotions.

Scientific studies on pregnancy cravings have consistently shown that there is no link between cravings and the baby's gender. Cravings are a normal part of pregnancy for many women, but they are influenced by a variety of factors that have nothing to do with whether the baby is a boy or a girl. In fact, some women report having different cravings with each pregnancy, regardless of the baby's gender.

While cravings can be a fun topic of conversation, they should not be used as a method of gender prediction. Instead, cravings should be viewed as a natural response to the body's changing needs during pregnancy. Expectant mothers can satisfy their cravings in moderation while ensuring that they maintain a balanced and nutritious diet that supports both their health and the health of their baby.

Evidence-Based Insights into Gender Determination

While old wives' tales and myths about gender prediction can be entertaining, they are not based on scientific evidence. Fortunately, modern medical science offers several accurate and reliable methods for determining the gender of a baby during pregnancy. These methods are based on an examination of the baby's chromosomes or anatomy, providing expectant parents with a clear and definitive answer about their baby's gender.

One of the most common and widely used methods for gender determination is the ultrasound. Ultrasound technology allows healthcare providers to visualize the baby's anatomy, including the genitalia, which can reveal the baby's gender. The optimal time for determining gender through ultrasound is typically around 18 to 20 weeks of pregnancy, during the second trimester. At this stage, the baby's genitalia are usually developed enough to be visible on the ultrasound image. However, factors such as the baby's position or the quality of the ultrasound equipment can sometimes make it difficult to get a clear view.

In addition to ultrasounds, there are more advanced and earlier methods for determining a baby's gender with even greater accuracy. One such method is Non-Invasive Prenatal Testing (NIPT), which has become increasingly popular in recent years. NIPT is a blood test that can be performed as early as 10 weeks into pregnancy. It analyzes small fragments of fetal DNA that circulate in the mother's bloodstream. This test is primarily used to screen for chromosomal abnormalities, such as Down syndrome, but it can also determine the baby's gender with a high degree of accuracy by identifying the presence or absence of the Y chromosome. If Y chromosomes are detected, the baby is male; if not, the baby is female.

NIPT has a very high accuracy rate, typically greater than 99% for gender determination, and carries no risk to the mother or baby since it is non-invasive. However, it is important to note that NIPT is a screening test, not a diagnostic test, meaning that it provides highly accurate results but is not a 100% guarantee.

Another method of determining the baby's gender is amniocentesis, a diagnostic procedure that involves collecting a sample of amniotic fluid from around the baby. Amniocentesis is usually performed between 15 and 20 weeks of pregnancy and is used to diagnose chromosomal abnormalities and genetic disorders. Because the baby's DNA is present in the amniotic fluid, the test can also determine the baby's gender. While amniocentesis is very accurate, it is an invasive procedure and carries a small risk of complications, including miscarriage. Therefore, it is typically only recommended when there is a medical indication, such as a higher risk of genetic disorders, rather than for gender determination alone.

Chorionic villus sampling (CVS) is another invasive diagnostic test that can determine the baby's gender. CVS is usually performed between 10 and 13 weeks of pregnancy and involves collecting a small sample of tissue from the placenta. Like amniocentesis, CVS is used to diagnose genetic conditions and can also reveal the baby's gender with a high degree of accuracy. However, because CVS is invasive and carries a small risk of complications, it is generally only recommended for specific medical reasons.

It is important to recognize that while modern medical science provides accurate methods for determining a baby's gender, the ability to find out the gender before birth is a relatively recent development. For centuries, parents relied on myths, old wives' tales, and personal observations to guess the gender of their baby. Even today, with access to advanced medical testing, some parents choose to engage in these gender prediction traditions as part of the fun and excitement of pregnancy.

However, it is essential to approach these myths with an understanding that they are not based on science. While guessing the baby's gender based on belly shape, heart rate, or cravings may be entertaining, expectant parents should not rely on these methods for accurate information. Instead, they should turn to evidence-based medical tests if they wish to know their baby's gender before birth.

For some parents, waiting until the birth to find out the baby's gender is a deliberate choice. The element of surprise can add to the excitement and anticipation of the delivery day. In such cases, focusing on the health and well-being of both the mother and the baby is the priority, rather than getting caught up in gender prediction myths. Ultimately, whether parents choose to find out their baby's gender early through medical testing or wait until birth, the most important factor is that the baby is healthy.

In conclusion, while old wives' tales and myths about gender prediction remain popular in many cultures, they are not reliable methods for determining a baby's gender. The shape of the belly, the baby's heart rate, and food cravings are influenced by a variety of factors unrelated to the baby's gender. Modern medical science offers accurate and non-invasive methods, such as ultrasounds and NIPT, as well as invasive procedures like amniocentesis and CVS, to determine the baby's gender with high accuracy. Expectant parents should rely on these evidence-based methods if they wish to know their baby's gender, while keeping in mind that the health and happiness of both the baby and the mother are the ultimate priorities during pregnancy.

Nutrition and Cravings Myths

Pregnancy is a time of significant physical and emotional changes, and these changes often manifest in a heightened focus on nutrition. The common adage that "you are what you eat" takes on new meaning for expectant mothers, as they are now not only responsible for their own health but also for the developing life inside them. This heightened awareness of nutrition during pregnancy has, however, been clouded by a variety of myths and misconceptions. Some of these myths are deeply ingrained in cultural traditions, while others have emerged from a misunderstanding of scientific facts. In this chapter, we will address three prevalent myths about pregnancy nutrition—"eating for two," indulging in cravings, and avoiding seafood—and then explore the evidence-based truth about maintaining a balanced and healthy diet during pregnancy.

Myth 7: You Need to Eat for Two

One of the most widely believed and persistent myths surrounding pregnancy is the notion that expectant mothers need to "eat for two." This phrase suggests that a pregnant woman must double her food intake to provide adequate nutrition for herself and her baby. While this myth has been passed down through generations, it is not only misleading but also potentially harmful. The truth is that while a pregnant woman's nutritional needs do increase, the amount of food required is far from doubling.

The origins of this myth likely stem from the fact that pregnant women do indeed need to consume additional nutrients to support the growth and development of the fetus. However, the actual caloric increase is far less dramatic than the idea of "eating for two" suggests. According to the American College of Obstetricians and Gynecologists (ACOG), most pregnant women only need an additional 300 to 450 calories per day during the second and third trimesters. To put this into perspective, 300 to 450 calories is equivalent to a small snack, such as a piece of whole-grain toast with peanut butter or a cup of yogurt with fruit. This is a far cry from doubling one's daily caloric intake.

In the first trimester, most women do not need to consume any additional calories at all. During the early stages of pregnancy, the baby is very small, and the mother's body is still adjusting to the hormonal and metabolic changes that accompany pregnancy. The focus during the first trimester should be on consuming nutrient-dense foods that provide essential vitamins and minerals, rather than increasing caloric intake.

It is important to recognize that excessive weight gain during pregnancy can lead to complications for both the mother and the baby. Overeating in response to the "eating for two" myth can contribute to excessive weight gain, which increases the risk of gestational diabetes, hypertension, and complications during labor and delivery. Additionally, excessive weight gain during pregnancy can make it more difficult for a woman to return to her pre-pregnancy weight after childbirth, potentially leading to long-term health issues such as obesity and cardiovascular disease.

On the other hand, under-eating or severely restricting calories during pregnancy can also be harmful. A pregnant woman's body requires a variety of nutrients, including protein, healthy fats, vitamins, and minerals, to support both her health and the development of her baby. Failing to meet these nutritional needs can result in poor fetal growth, low birth weight, and developmental problems. It is essential for pregnant women to strike a balance by eating enough to meet their increased nutritional needs without overindulging.

The key to healthy eating during pregnancy is not about eating for two, but rather about focusing on the quality of the food being consumed. Nutrient-dense foods, such as fruits, vegetables, whole grains, lean proteins, and healthy fats, provide the essential nutrients that both the mother and the baby need. By choosing foods that are rich in vitamins, minerals, and other important nutrients, pregnant women can support their health and the health of their developing baby without consuming excessive calories.

Myth 8: All Pregnancy Cravings Should Be Indulged

Pregnancy cravings are a well-known phenomenon, and many women experience intense desires for specific foods during pregnancy. Cravings can range from the typical (chocolate, ice cream, salty snacks) to the unusual (pickles and peanut butter, or chalk). While cravings are a normal part of pregnancy, the idea that all cravings should be indulged without consideration of nutritional value is a myth that can lead to unhealthy eating habits and potential complications.

Cravings during pregnancy are thought to be influenced by a variety of factors, including hormonal changes, nutrient deficiencies, and emotional or psychological factors. For example, some women may crave salty foods because their body needs more sodium, or they may crave sweets when their blood sugar levels drop. Hormonal fluctuations during pregnancy, particularly the rise in estrogen and progesterone, can also affect taste and smell, making certain foods more appealing or unappealing.

While occasional indulgence in cravings is not inherently harmful, the belief that all cravings should be satisfied without restriction can lead to poor dietary choices. Many common pregnancy cravings, such as sweets, processed snacks, and fast food, are high in sugar, unhealthy fats, and sodium. Regularly indulging in these types of foods can contribute to excessive weight gain, gestational diabetes, and other pregnancy-related complications.

Gestational diabetes, a condition characterized by high blood sugar levels during pregnancy, is a particular concern for women who frequently indulge in sugary cravings. Women with gestational diabetes are at higher risk of developing type 2 diabetes later in life, and their babies are at increased risk of being born with a higher birth weight, which can lead to complications during delivery. Additionally, babies born to mothers with gestational diabetes are more likely to develop obesity and metabolic disorders later in life.

It is also important to address the issue of non-food cravings, known as pica, which is the craving for substances that are not food, such as dirt, clay, or laundry starch. Pica can be dangerous, as consuming non-food items can lead to poisoning, infections, or nutritional deficiencies. Women who experience cravings for non-food substances should consult their healthcare provider to address any underlying nutrient deficiencies or health concerns.

Rather than indulging in all cravings without consideration, pregnant women should focus on finding healthier alternatives that satisfy their cravings while providing essential nutrients. For example, if a woman craves something sweet, she can choose fruit, yogurt, or a small portion of dark chocolate instead of sugary candy or baked goods. If she craves something salty, she can opt for lightly salted nuts, air-popped popcorn, or whole-grain crackers instead of processed chips or fast food. By making mindful choices, women can satisfy their cravings while still maintaining a healthy and balanced diet.

It is also helpful for pregnant women to pay attention to their body's signals and identify the root cause of their cravings. For example, if a woman is craving sweets, it may be because her blood sugar levels are low, and she can address this by eating a balanced meal or snack that includes complex carbohydrates, protein, and healthy fats. If a woman is craving salty foods, it may be because her body needs more sodium or electrolytes, and she can meet this need by incorporating nutrient-rich foods such as avocado, nuts, or whole grains into her diet.

In conclusion, while cravings are a normal part of pregnancy, not all cravings should be indulged without consideration of their nutritional impact. Pregnant women should focus on finding healthier alternatives that satisfy their cravings while supporting their health and the health of their baby. By maintaining a balanced and mindful approach to eating, women can enjoy their pregnancy cravings in moderation without compromising their overall nutrition.

Myth 9: You Can't Eat Seafood During Pregnancy

Seafood is often the subject of confusion and concern for pregnant women, leading to the widespread belief that seafood should be completely avoided during pregnancy. This myth likely stems from concerns about mercury contamination and foodborne illnesses associated with certain types of fish. While it is true that pregnant women should be cautious about their seafood choices, the blanket avoidance of all seafood is both unnecessary and detrimental to maternal and fetal health.

Seafood, particularly fish, is an excellent source of high-quality protein, omega-3 fatty acids (especially DHA and EPA), vitamins, and minerals such as iodine and selenium. Omega-3 fatty acids, in particular, play a crucial role in the development of the baby's brain and eyes. Numerous studies have shown that pregnant women who consume adequate amounts of omega-3s from fish and seafood have babies with better cognitive and visual development.

The primary concern with seafood during pregnancy is the potential exposure to high levels of mercury, a toxic metal that can harm the developing nervous system of the fetus. Mercury is found in varying levels in different types of fish, and the highest concentrations are typically found in large predatory fish such as shark, swordfish, king mackerel, and tile fish. Because these fish are at the top of the food chain, they accumulate higher levels of mercury in their bodies over time.

However, many types of seafood are low in mercury and are safe for pregnant women to eat in moderation. The U.S. Food and Drug Administration (FDA) and the Environmental Protection Agency (EPA) recommend that pregnant women consume 8 to 12 ounces (about two to three servings) of low-mercury seafood per week. Safe options include salmon, sardines, trout, anchovies, shrimp, crab, and tilapia. These fish provide essential nutrients without posing a significant risk of mercury exposure.

In addition to mercury concerns, pregnant women are often advised to avoid raw or under-cooked seafood, such as sushi or oysters, due to the risk of foodborne illnesses caused by bacteria, parasites, or viruses. Listeria, in particular, is a type of bacteria that can contaminate certain foods, including raw or smoked seafood, and can lead to miscarriage, premature birth, or stillbirth. To minimize the risk of foodborne illness, pregnant women should avoid raw or under-cooked seafood and opt for cooked seafood instead.

It is important to note that the benefits of consuming low-mercury seafood during pregnancy far outweigh the risks. The omega-3 fatty acids found in fish, especially DHA and EPA, are crucial for the baby's brain and eye development. Studies have shown that babies born to mothers who consume adequate amounts of omega-3s during pregnancy tend to have better cognitive and visual outcomes. Additionally, seafood provides essential nutrients like iodine, selenium, and vitamin D, all of which are important for both maternal health and fetal development. Iodine, for instance, plays a critical role in regulating the mother's thyroid function, which is essential for fetal brain development.

To strike a balance between the benefits and risks of seafood consumption during pregnancy, it is important for expectant mothers to be mindful of their choices. Low-mercury fish, such as salmon, sardines, and trout, can be consumed safely and offer the necessary nutrients that benefit both mother and baby. Pregnant women should avoid high-mercury fish like shark, swordfish, king mackerel, and tile fish, but they do not need to avoid seafood altogether. Moderation is key, and by choosing low-mercury, nutrient-rich seafood, pregnant women can support the healthy development of their baby while minimizing potential risks.

In summary, the belief that all seafood must be avoided during pregnancy is a myth. While certain high-mercury fish should be avoided, many types of seafood are safe and beneficial for pregnant women. By focusing on low-mercury options and ensuring that seafood is cooked thoroughly, women can enjoy the health benefits of fish and seafood without undue concern about mercury exposure or foodborne illnesses. Seafood can and should be part of a balanced, nutritious diet during pregnancy, as it provides essential nutrients that are important for both maternal and fetal health.

Truth About Pregnancy Nutrition and How to Maintain a Balanced Diet

Pregnancy is a time when proper nutrition is more important than ever, as the food a mother consumes directly impacts both her health and the health of her developing baby. However, the abundance of myths and conflicting information about pregnancy nutrition can make it difficult for expectant mothers to know what they should eat and what they should avoid. In this section, we will explore the evidence-based truth about pregnancy nutrition and provide practical tips for maintaining a balanced, healthy diet during pregnancy.

One of the most important aspects of pregnancy nutrition is ensuring that the mother is consuming enough of the essential nutrients needed to support the baby's growth and development. These include key nutrients like folic acid, iron, calcium, omega-3 fatty acids, protein, and a wide variety of vitamins and minerals. A well-balanced diet that includes a variety of nutrient-dense foods can help meet these nutritional needs and promote a healthy pregnancy.

Folic Acid: Folic acid, or folate, is one of the most critical nutrients during pregnancy, especially in the early stages. It helps prevent neural tube defects (NTDs), which are serious birth defects of the brain and spine, such as spina bifida. Pregnant women are advised to take a prenatal vitamin that contains at least 400 to 800 micrograms of folic acid daily, in addition to consuming foods that are rich in folate, such as leafy green vegetables, citrus fruits, and fortified grains.

Iron: Iron is another essential nutrient during pregnancy, as it helps produce the extra blood needed to supply oxygen to the baby. Many pregnant women are at risk of iron deficiency anemia, which can lead to fatigue and increase the risk of preterm birth or low birth weight. Iron-rich foods include red meat, poultry, beans, lentils, spinach, and fortified cereals. It is also helpful to pair iron-rich foods with vitamin C-rich foods, such as oranges or bell peppers, to enhance iron absorption.

Calcium: Calcium is important for the development of the baby's bones and teeth. Pregnant women need around 1,000 milligrams of calcium per day to support their own bone health and the growing baby's needs. Dairy products like milk, yogurt, and cheese are excellent sources of calcium, but it can also be found in fortified plant-based milks, leafy greens, and tofu.

Omega-3 Fatty Acids: As mentioned earlier, omega-3 fatty acids, particularly DHA and EPA, are crucial for the development of the baby's brain and eyes. Pregnant women should aim to consume at least 200 to 300 milligrams of DHA daily, which can be found in fatty fish like salmon, sardines, and trout, as well as in fortified foods and supplements. Omega-3s not only support fetal development but also have been shown to reduce the risk of preterm birth and improve maternal mental health.

Protein: Protein is the building block of cells and tissues, and it plays a vital role in the baby's growth and development. Pregnant women should aim to consume around 70 to 100 grams of protein per day, depending on their individual needs. Good sources of protein include lean meats, poultry, fish, eggs, beans, lentils, tofu, and dairy products. Protein-rich snacks, such as Greek yogurt or a handful of nuts, can also help meet daily protein requirements.

Fruits and Vegetables: A varied intake of fruits and vegetables is essential for providing the vitamins, minerals, and fiber needed during pregnancy. These foods are rich in antioxidants, which help protect the mother and baby from oxidative stress, and they provide essential nutrients like vitamin C, potassium, and fiber. Pregnant women should aim to fill half their plate with fruits and vegetables at each meal, choosing a variety of colors to ensure they are getting a wide range of nutrients.

Whole Grains: Whole grains, such as brown rice, quinoa, oats, and whole wheat bread, provide important nutrients like fiber, B vitamins, and magnesium. These grains help maintain steady blood sugar levels, provide energy, and support digestive health, which can be especially important during pregnancy when constipation is a common issue. Pregnant women should aim to include whole grains in their daily meals to support overall health and provide sustained energy.

Hydration: Staying hydrated is crucial during pregnancy, as the body requires extra fluids to support the increased blood volume and amniotic fluid. Pregnant women should aim to drink at least 8 to 10 cups of water per day, and more if they are physically active or experiencing symptoms like nausea or vomiting. Staying well-hydrated can also help prevent common pregnancy discomforts like constipation and swelling.

While it's important to focus on nutrient-dense foods, pregnancy is not a time for extreme diets or restrictive eating. Pregnant women should aim to meet their nutritional needs through a variety of whole foods while allowing themselves occasional treats in moderation. The key is balance—ensuring that the majority of the diet consists of healthy, nutrient-rich foods, while still enjoying favorite foods in a mindful and moderate way.

Managing Common Pregnancy Nutrition Challenges:

Pregnancy can bring about various challenges related to nutrition, such as morning sickness, food aversions, and changes in appetite. For women experiencing morning sickness or nausea, it can be helpful to eat small, frequent meals throughout the day and choose bland, easily digestible foods like crackers, toast, or bananas. Ginger and peppermint tea are also known to help alleviate nausea. Women who experience food aversions can try incorporating alternative sources of essential nutrients if certain foods become unappealing. For example, if meat is difficult to tolerate, they can opt for plant-based protein sources like beans, lentils, or tofu.

Some women may also struggle with heartburn or indigestion, especially in the later stages of pregnancy. To reduce these symptoms, it is recommended to eat smaller meals, avoid spicy or fatty foods, and stay upright for a while after eating. Additionally, pregnant women should avoid lying down immediately after meals and should aim to eat their last meal of the day several hours before bedtime.

In conclusion, maintaining a balanced and nutritious diet during pregnancy is essential for both the mother's health and the baby's development. While many myths persist about pregnancy nutrition, the evidence-based truth is that expectant mothers do not need to "eat for two," should be mindful about indulging cravings, and can safely enjoy seafood by choosing low-mercury options. By focusing on nutrient-dense foods and meeting the body's increased nutritional needs, pregnant women can support a healthy pregnancy and give their baby the best possible start in life.

Physical Activity and Exercise Myths

During pregnancy, physical activity and exercise are often sources of confusion and concern for expectant mothers. While pregnancy brings about significant changes in a woman's body, many of which can be physically demanding, there are persistent myths surrounding the idea of whether and how exercise should be part of an expectant mother's routine. These myths, often rooted in outdated beliefs or misunderstandings, can discourage pregnant women from engaging in beneficial physical activity. On the other hand, staying active during pregnancy has been shown to provide a wide range of health benefits for both mother and baby. In this chapter, we will address three common myths related to pregnancy and exercise—avoiding exercise, concerns about running, and the dangers of weightlifting—and provide clear, evidence-based guidelines for maintaining a safe and healthy fitness routine throughout pregnancy.

Myth 10: Pregnant Women Should Avoid Exercise

One of the most pervasive myths about pregnancy is that women should avoid exercise altogether for fear that it may harm the baby or cause complications. For many years, this belief was commonly accepted, with the idea that pregnant women should "take it easy" and avoid exerting themselves physically. However, modern research has thoroughly debunked this myth, showing that regular physical activity is not only safe for most pregnant women but also highly beneficial for both maternal and fetal health.

The origins of this myth likely stem from the historical treatment of pregnancy as a fragile or delicate condition, where women were often advised to rest and avoid physical strain. However, pregnancy is a natural and dynamic state, not a sickness, and most women can continue to engage in physical activity throughout their pregnancy as long as they follow appropriate guidelines and consult with their healthcare providers. In fact, the American College of Obstetricians and Gynecologists (ACOG) recommends that pregnant women engage in at least 150 minutes of moderate-intensity aerobic activity per week, which is similar to the recommendations for the general population.

The benefits of exercise during pregnancy are numerous. Regular physical activity helps improve cardiovascular health, increase muscle tone, and support healthy weight gain during pregnancy. It also helps alleviate common pregnancy discomforts such as back pain, constipation, and swelling, and it can improve energy levels, mood, and sleep. Additionally, staying active during pregnancy can help reduce the risk of gestational diabetes, preeclampsia, and other pregnancy-related complications. For the baby, maternal exercise has been associated with a reduced risk of excessive birth weight and improved fetal heart health.

Furthermore, physical activity during pregnancy can help prepare a woman's body for the physical demands of labor and delivery. Childbirth is an intense physical event, and having a strong cardiovascular system, toned muscles, and good endurance can aid in the process. Women who maintain regular physical activity throughout their pregnancy may experience shorter labor times and reduced need for interventions such as epidurals or cesarean deliveries.

Of course, there are some instances where certain types of exercise may need to be modified or avoided due to medical conditions or complications. For example, women with placenta previa, preterm labor risk, or severe preeclampsia should avoid strenuous activities and follow their healthcare provider's guidance. However, for most pregnant women, physical activity can and should be a part of their daily routine, as long as it is done safely and with proper consideration of the body's changing needs.

In conclusion, the idea that pregnant women should avoid exercise is an outdated and inaccurate myth. For most women, regular physical activity during pregnancy is not only safe but also beneficial for both mother and baby. Expectant mothers should consult with their healthcare providers to determine the best exercise routine for their individual needs, but they should feel confident in staying active throughout their pregnancy.

Myth 11: Running Can Cause Miscarriage

Running, one of the most popular forms of exercise, is often surrounded by myths when it comes to pregnancy. One of the most alarming misconceptions is that running during pregnancy can cause miscarriage, especially in the early stages. This myth has caused unnecessary fear for many women, leading them to stop running or avoid it altogether during pregnancy. However, there is no scientific evidence to support the idea that running can cause miscarriage in a healthy pregnancy.

Miscarriage is a deeply emotional and often misunderstood event, and it is natural for women to be cautious about potential causes. However, most miscarriages occur due to chromosomal abnormalities or other factors unrelated to physical activity. Running, when done safely and with appropriate precautions, does not increase the risk of miscarriage in a normal, healthy pregnancy.

In fact, many women who were runners before becoming pregnant can safely continue running throughout their pregnancy, provided they listen to their bodies and make any necessary adjustments as their pregnancy progresses. The key is moderation and paying attention to how the body responds to the activity. For example, some women may find that as their pregnancy progresses, they need to reduce their intensity or switch to lower-impact activities such as swimming or walking. However, for those who are comfortable continuing to run, there is no need to fear that it will cause harm to the baby.

It is also important to note that many elite and recreational athletes have continued to run throughout their pregnancies without any adverse effects. Serena Williams, for example, famously competed in tennis tournaments while pregnant, and many long-distance runners have completed races while expecting. These examples demonstrate that the body is capable of adapting to physical activity during pregnancy, provided that the woman listens to her body's signals and adjusts as needed.

That said, there are some precautions that pregnant runners should take to ensure their safety. As the pregnancy progresses, the body's center of gravity shifts, which can affect balance and increase the risk of falls. Running on flat, even surfaces and avoiding rough or uneven terrain can help reduce this risk. Staying hydrated is also crucial, as pregnant women are more prone to dehydration. Wearing supportive shoes and comfortable, breathable clothing can further enhance comfort and safety during runs.

As with any exercise, it is important for pregnant women to consult with their healthcare provider before continuing or starting a running routine. For women with certain pregnancy complications, such as placenta previa or a history of preterm labor, running may not be advisable. However, for most women with uncomplicated pregnancies, running is a safe and effective form of exercise.

In conclusion, the myth that running can cause miscarriage is not supported by scientific evidence. For women with healthy pregnancies, running can be a safe and beneficial form of physical activity. As long as expectant mothers listen to their bodies, make necessary adjustments, and consult with their healthcare providers, they can continue to enjoy running throughout their pregnancy without fear of harm to themselves or their babies.

Myth 12: Lifting Weights is Dangerous for Pregnant Women

Another common misconception about pregnancy and exercise is that lifting weights is inherently dangerous for pregnant women. Many people believe that weightlifting can strain the body, harm the baby, or lead to complications such as preterm labor or miscarriage. While it is true that certain modifications may be necessary during pregnancy, the idea that pregnant women should completely avoid weightlifting is a myth.

In reality, strength training, when done properly, can be a safe and effective way to maintain muscle tone, improve posture, and support overall fitness during pregnancy. In fact, maintaining muscle strength can help reduce the risk of injury, improve balance, and alleviate common pregnancy discomforts such as back pain. Strong muscles also play a critical role in supporting the pelvic floor, which is essential for labor and delivery.

The key to safe weightlifting during pregnancy is to modify the exercises as needed and avoid overexertion. As the pregnancy progresses, women may need to reduce the amount of weight they lift, increase their focus on proper form, and avoid exercises that involve lying flat on the back or lifting heavy weights overhead. It is also important to avoid exercises that place excessive strain on the abdominal muscles, as this can increase the risk of diastasis recti (the separation of the abdominal muscles).

Pregnant women who are new to weightlifting should start with light weights and focus on low-impact, controlled movements. It is essential to pay attention to the body's signals and stop immediately if any discomfort, dizziness, or shortness of breath occurs. Using resistance bands, body weight exercises, or lighter free weights can be excellent alternatives for maintaining strength without placing undue strain on the body.

For women who were already accustomed to weightlifting before becoming pregnant, continuing a modified strength training routine is generally safe as long as they follow appropriate guidelines and work with their healthcare provider to ensure they are exercising within their body's limits. Strengthening the muscles of the legs, arms, back, and core can provide significant benefits during pregnancy, labor, and postpartum recovery.

It is also important to dispel the myth that weightlifting can lead to miscarriage or preterm labor. As with running, the vast majority of miscarriages are caused by genetic or chromosomal abnormalities, not by physical activity. Studies have shown that moderate strength training during pregnancy is safe and does not increase the risk of preterm labor in healthy pregnancies. In fact, staying active and maintaining muscle strength can reduce the risk of complications such as excessive weight gain, gestational diabetes, and hypertension.

In conclusion, weightlifting is not inherently dangerous for pregnant women, and in many cases, it can be a valuable part of a prenatal fitness routine. By making appropriate modifications, focusing on proper form, and listening to their bodies, expectant mothers can safely engage in strength training throughout pregnancy. As always, it is essential to consult with a healthcare provider to ensure that any exercise routine is safe and appropriate for an individual's specific circumstances.

Safe Exercise Guidelines for Expecting Moms

While exercise during pregnancy is generally safe and beneficial, it is important to follow certain guidelines to ensure that physical activity is done safely. Every pregnancy is unique, and it is essential for expectant mothers to work with their healthcare providers to develop an exercise plan that meets their individual needs. Here are some evidence-based guidelines to help pregnant women maintain a safe and effective fitness routine:

1. Consult with a Healthcare Provider: Before starting or continuing any exercise routine during pregnancy, it is crucial to get approval from a

healthcare provider. This step ensures that the expectant mother's specific health needs, potential complications, and fitness levels are taken into consideration. Women with certain conditions, such as placenta previa, a history of preterm labor, or high blood pressure, may need to avoid or modify their exercise routines. However, most women with uncomplicated pregnancies can safely engage in regular physical activity.

2. Aim for 150 Minutes of Moderate Exercise Per Week: According to guidelines from the American College of Obstetricians and Gynecologists (ACOG), pregnant women should aim for at least 150 minutes of moderate-intensity aerobic activity per week. This can be broken down into 30-minute sessions on most days of the week. Moderate-intensity exercise includes activities like brisk walking, swimming, stationary cycling, or prenatal yoga. During moderate exercise, a woman should be able to talk but not sing, indicating that she is working at an appropriate intensity level.

3. Choose Low-Impact Activities: Low-impact exercises are ideal for pregnancy, as they reduce the risk of injury and minimize stress on the joints and ligaments, which become more flexible due to the hormone relaxing. Walking, swimming, stationary biking, and prenatal yoga are excellent low-impact options. Swimming, in particular, is often recommended because it provides a full-body workout while being easy on the joints, and the buoyancy of the water helps alleviate the strain of carrying extra weight.

4. Stay Hydrated: Pregnant women are more prone to dehydration, which can increase the risk of overheating and other complications. It is essential to drink plenty of water before, during, and after exercise. Women should also avoid exercising in hot, humid conditions to reduce the risk of overheating and dehydration.

5. Listen to Your Body: Pregnancy is a time when the body undergoes significant changes, and it is important for expectant mothers to pay close attention to how their bodies feel during exercise. If a woman experiences

any dizziness, shortness of breath, chest pain, uterine contractions, vaginal bleeding, or severe discomfort, she should stop exercising immediately and seek medical attention. Exercise should always feel challenging but not painful or overwhelming.

6. Avoid Exercises that Involve Lying Flat on the Back After the First Trimester: After the first trimester, exercises that involve lying flat on the back, such as some Pilates or yoga positions, should be avoided. Lying on the back can compress the inferior vena cava, a major vein that carries blood from the lower body to the heart, potentially causing dizziness, low blood pressure, or reduced blood flow to the baby. Instead, women can modify exercises by performing them in a side-lying, standing, or seated position.

7. Be Mindful of Balance and Stability: As pregnancy progresses, the growing belly shifts a woman's center of gravity, which can affect balance and increase the risk of falls. Activities that require good balance, such as biking or running on uneven terrain, may become more challenging. To minimize the risk of injury, pregnant women should focus on exercises that provide stability, such as walking on flat surfaces, using a stationary bike, or performing strength training exercises with the support of a chair or wall.

8. Incorporate Strength Training: Strength training can be a valuable component of a prenatal fitness routine, as it helps build and maintain muscle strength, improve posture, and support overall physical health. Pregnant women should focus on exercises that strengthen the legs, back, and core, which can help alleviate common pregnancy discomforts and prepare the body for labor. Light to moderate weights, resistance bands, or bodyweight exercises are excellent options. However, it is important to avoid heavy lifting or exercises that strain the abdominal muscles.

9. Modify Exercises as Needed: As the pregnancy progresses, certain exercises may need to be modified to accommodate the growing belly and changing body. Women may need to reduce the intensity, switch to lower-impact

activities, or avoid exercises that cause discomfort. Prenatal yoga or Pilates classes, which are specifically designed for pregnant women, can provide safe, effective workouts that focus on strength, flexibility, and relaxation.

10. Cool Down and Stretch After Exercise: After completing a workout, it is important to take time to cool down and stretch. Stretching helps improve flexibility, relieve tension, and prevent muscle soreness. Gentle stretching exercises, particularly for the back, hips, and legs, can help alleviate common pregnancy aches and pains. Additionally, prenatal yoga classes often incorporate stretching and relaxation techniques that can be beneficial for both physical and mental well-being.

11. Avoid Contact Sports and High-Risk Activities: Pregnant women should avoid contact sports and activities that carry a high risk of falling or injury, such as horseback riding, skiing, or mountain biking. These activities can increase the risk of trauma to both the mother and the baby. Additionally, scuba diving should be avoided during pregnancy due to the risk of decompression sickness, which can affect the baby.

12. Don't Overdo It: While regular exercise is important, it is equally important not to overexert oneself during pregnancy. Pregnancy is not the time to set new fitness goals or push the body to its limits. The goal of exercise during pregnancy should be to maintain overall health, manage weight gain, and support physical and mental well-being. Women should avoid intense or prolonged workouts that leave them feeling exhausted or unable to recover quickly.

13. Stay Mentally Engaged: Exercise during pregnancy is not just about physical fitness; it also has mental and emotional benefits. Physical activity can help reduce stress, anxiety, and depression, which are common during pregnancy. Mind-body exercises such as yoga, meditation, or deep breathing can help promote relaxation and mental clarity, which can be especially helpful during the challenges of pregnancy.

In conclusion, staying active during pregnancy offers numerous health benefits for both the mother and the baby. By following these safe exercise guidelines, pregnant women can maintain their fitness, improve their physical and mental well-being, and prepare their bodies for labor and postpartum recovery. While myths about pregnancy and exercise persist, the evidence shows that physical activity, when done safely, is a valuable tool for promoting a healthy pregnancy. Expectant mothers should feel confident in their ability to stay active throughout pregnancy, as long as they listen to their bodies and consult with their healthcare providers to develop a safe and effective exercise routine tailored to their individual needs.

Medical Myths

Pregnancy is a time filled with anticipation and excitement, but it is also often accompanied by a flood of information, much of which can be misleading or incorrect. The internet, well-meaning friends and family members, and even cultural traditions can perpetuate myths that shape a pregnant woman's expectations and decision-making. Among the most critical areas where myths can cause confusion is in medical interventions and health practices during pregnancy. These myths not only create unnecessary anxiety but can also lead to decisions that are not in the best interest of the mother or baby. In this chapter, we will explore some of the most common medical myths that pregnant women encounter, specifically those related to cesarean sections (C-sections), the notion that all pregnancies are the same, and the misconception about avoiding all medications. Additionally, we will look at what you should be asking your doctor to get accurate, evidence-based information about medical interventions.

Myth 13: C-Sections Are the "Easy Way Out"

One of the most pervasive myths surrounding childbirth is the idea that cesarean sections (C-sections) are an "easy way out" for women. This myth often carries with it a sense of judgment, suggesting that women who undergo a C-section are choosing to avoid the challenges of labor and delivery. However, the reality of C-sections is far from easy, and this misconception can diminish the very real physical and emotional toll that such a procedure can take on a woman.

A C-section is a major surgical procedure in which an incision is made through the mother's abdomen and uterus to deliver the baby. It is typically performed when a vaginal birth would pose a risk to the mother or baby's health, such as in cases of fetal distress, breech presentation, or placental complications. In some cases, it may be planned in advance due to medical conditions, while in others, it may be decided in an emergency situation when labor is not progressing as expected or complications arise.

While C-sections are sometimes medically necessary and can be life-saving, they are by no means an "easy" option. The recovery period for a C-section is generally longer and more challenging than for a vaginal birth. Women who undergo a C-section often experience more pain and discomfort in the weeks following the surgery, and they are at greater risk for complications such as infections, blood clots, and longer hospital stays. Additionally, the emotional aspect of having a C-section, particularly if it was unplanned or the result of an emergency, can be difficult for some women to process. The feeling of losing control over their birth plan or experiencing a surgical birth instead of a vaginal delivery can lead to disappointment or even postpartum depression.

It is important to acknowledge that the decision to have a C-section is not one that women take lightly. In many cases, the procedure is performed to ensure the safest possible outcome for both mother and baby. While some women may feel relief at the prospect of avoiding a prolonged labor, the physical and emotional challenges of a C-section should not be underestimated. This myth perpetuates a harmful narrative that dismisses the legitimate medical reasons for a C-section and undermines the experiences of women who undergo this major surgery.

Rather than viewing C-sections as the "easy way out," it is essential to recognize them as a necessary medical intervention in certain circumstances. Every woman's childbirth experience is unique, and there is no single "right" way to give birth. Whether through vaginal delivery or C-section, the ultimate goal is a safe and healthy outcome for both mother and baby.

Myth 14: Every Pregnancy Is the Same

Another common myth that often influences women's expectations during pregnancy is the belief that every pregnancy is the same. This misconception can lead to unrealistic comparisons between pregnancies, both within the same woman's experiences and between different women. While there are certainly commonalities in the physiological processes of pregnancy, each pregnancy is a unique experience shaped by a variety of factors, including genetics, maternal health, environmental influences, and individual circumstances.

Many women who have experienced multiple pregnancies can attest to the fact that no two pregnancies are alike. Some women may have relatively easy pregnancies with minimal discomfort, while others may struggle with more severe symptoms such as morning sickness, fatigue, or back pain. Even within the same woman, one pregnancy may be vastly different from another. A woman who had a smooth, complication-free pregnancy the first time around may face unexpected challenges in a subsequent pregnancy, or vice versa.

This myth can create unnecessary stress and self-doubt, particularly for women who feel that their pregnancy is not "normal" compared to others. For example, a woman who experiences debilitating morning sickness in her first pregnancy may feel discouraged if she expected her second pregnancy to be easier, based on her previous experience. Alternatively, women may feel pressured to minimize their symptoms or concerns if they believe that pregnancy should be a uniform experience.

It is essential to understand that every pregnancy is influenced by a wide range of factors, many of which are outside of a woman's control. Maternal age, pre-existing health conditions, stress levels, nutrition, and even the baby's position in the womb can all affect how a pregnancy progresses. Additionally, advances in medical knowledge and prenatal care mean that some aspects of pregnancy management may change between pregnancies, further contributing to differences in the experience.

Rather than expecting every pregnancy to follow the same pattern, it is important for women to embrace the unique nature of each pregnancy and listen to their bodies. Open communication with healthcare providers is key to addressing any concerns or unexpected changes. By recognizing that no two pregnancies are the same, women can approach their pregnancy journey with greater flexibility and self-compassion, understanding that their experience is valid and does not need to conform to anyone else's.

Myth 15: You Should Avoid All Medications During Pregnancy

One of the most pervasive and potentially harmful myths about pregnancy is the idea that all medications should be avoided. While it is true that some medications can pose risks to a developing fetus, the blanket avoidance of all medications is neither necessary nor advisable in most cases. This myth can lead to unnecessary suffering for pregnant women who may need medications to manage chronic conditions, pain, or other health concerns, and it can also result in untreated medical issues that could pose a risk to both mother and baby.

The reality is that many medications are considered safe to use during pregnancy, and in some cases, they are essential for maintaining maternal health. Conditions such as asthma, diabetes, high blood pressure, and depression require ongoing management, and discontinuing necessary medications could lead to serious complications. For example, untreated high blood pressure during pregnancy can increase the risk of preeclampsia, a potentially life-threatening condition, while untreated asthma can reduce the amount of oxygen the baby receives.

The key to managing medication use during pregnancy is open communication with healthcare providers. Women should always inform their doctor or midwife about any medications they are taking, including over-the-counter medications, supplements, and herbal remedies. In many cases, healthcare providers can adjust the dosage, switch to a safer alternative, or provide guidance on how to manage symptoms without medication if appropriate. For example, certain medications used to treat depression or anxiety may need to be adjusted during pregnancy, but abruptly stopping these medications can be harmful to both the mother and baby. Healthcare providers can help women make informed decisions about the risks and benefits of continuing medication during pregnancy.

It is also important to note that there are certain medications that should be avoided during pregnancy due to the risk of birth defects or other complications. Nonsteroidal anti-inflammatory drugs (NSAIDs), such as ibuprofen and aspirin, are commonly advised against during pregnancy, especially in the later stages, as they can increase the risk of fetal and maternal complications, including premature closure of a blood vessel in the baby's heart (ductus arteriosus). Similarly, certain antibiotics, acne medications, and some herbal supplements may also pose risks to the developing fetus.

However, there are many other medications that are safe to use during pregnancy. For example, acetaminophen (Tylenol) is commonly recommended for pain relief and fever management. Some antibiotics, such as penicillin, are considered safe and necessary in treating infections during pregnancy. Prenatal vitamins, particularly those containing folic acid, are not only safe but essential for preventing neural tube defects and supporting the healthy development of the baby's brain and spine. Additionally, medications to manage chronic conditions, such as insulin for diabetes or antihypertensives for high blood pressure, are crucial for ensuring both maternal and fetal well-being.

One of the significant dangers of the "avoid all medications" myth is that it can lead women to forgo necessary treatments out of fear, potentially placing their health and their baby's health at risk. For example, untreated depression during pregnancy can increase the risk of preterm birth, low birth weight, and postpartum depression. Similarly, not managing chronic conditions like epilepsy or asthma with the appropriate medications can result in severe complications that could otherwise be prevented.

Therefore, it is essential for women to approach medication use during pregnancy with a nuanced perspective. The goal is not to avoid all medications, but rather to use them safely and judiciously under the guidance of a healthcare provider. By working closely with their doctor, pregnant women can navigate the potential risks and benefits of medications and make informed decisions that prioritize both their health and the health of their baby.

What to Ask Your Doctor: Facts About Medical Interventions

Pregnancy and childbirth come with a range of medical interventions, some planned and others potentially needed due to complications that arise during pregnancy or labor. Understanding the facts about these interventions, rather than relying on myths or misinformation, is crucial for making informed decisions. Whether it's about the possibility of a C-section, the use of medications, or any other medical interventions, open and honest communication with your healthcare provider is essential.

Here are key questions to ask your doctor to clarify facts about medical interventions and ensure that your choices are based on evidence and tailored to your individual needs:

1. When is a C-section necessary, and what should I expect during recovery?
   While C-sections are sometimes planned, they can also occur in emergency situations. It is essential to understand the medical reasons that may necessitate a C-section, such as fetal distress, breech presentation, or complications like placenta previa. By discussing these scenarios with your

doctor, you can gain a better understanding of when and why a C-section might be recommended. Additionally, asking about the recovery process, including potential complications, pain management, and postpartum care, will help you prepare mentally and physically for the possibility of a surgical birth.

2. How can I manage chronic health conditions during pregnancy?

If you have pre-existing health conditions such as diabetes, high blood pressure, or asthma, it's crucial to discuss how these conditions should be managed during pregnancy. Ask your doctor about the safety of continuing current medications and whether any adjustments need to be made. You should also inquire about how your condition may affect your pregnancy and what additional monitoring or interventions may be necessary to ensure the health of both you and your baby.

3. What medications are safe to use during pregnancy?

Pregnancy often brings new health concerns, such as morning sickness, heartburn, or pain, and you may wonder which medications are safe to use. Don't hesitate to ask your doctor about specific medications for common pregnancy symptoms, such as nausea, headaches, or allergies. If you're already taking medications for a chronic condition or mental health issue, clarify with your doctor whether it's safe to continue those medications or if alternatives should be considered.

4. What pain relief options are available during labor, and what are the risks and benefits?

Pain management during labor is a significant concern for many women, and there are various options available, ranging from natural methods to medical interventions such as epidurals or spinal anesthesia. Ask your doctor about the different types of pain relief, including the potential benefits and risks of each option. It's important to understand how these interventions might affect labor progression, as well as any potential side effects for both the mother and baby.

5. What can I do to prevent or manage pregnancy complications?

While it's impossible to predict every complication that may arise during pregnancy, there are steps you can take to reduce your risk. Talk to your doctor about any specific risk factors you may have, such as age, pre-existing conditions, or family history. Ask about preventive measures, such as appropriate weight gain, diet, exercise, and monitoring blood pressure or blood sugar levels. If complications do arise, such as gestational diabetes or preeclampsia, understanding the available treatments and interventions can help you manage these conditions and maintain a healthy pregnancy.

6. When should I consider medical interventions for labor induction or augmentation?

Induction of labor is sometimes necessary if the pregnancy goes past the due date, if there are concerns about the baby's growth, or if there are other medical reasons for expediting delivery. Ask your doctor about the conditions that may require induction and what methods are commonly used, such as medications or mechanical devices. You should also discuss the risks and benefits of inducing labor and whether there are any alternatives, such as waiting for labor to begin naturally.

7. What are the potential interventions during labor, and when might they be needed?

While most women hope for an uncomplicated labor and delivery, it's important to be prepared for the possibility of medical interventions. These may include the use of forceps or vacuum extraction, episiotomy (a surgical incision to enlarge the vaginal opening), or even an emergency C-section. Ask your doctor about the likelihood of needing these interventions, what signs might indicate they are necessary, and what you can expect if they are used. Understanding these possibilities in advance can help you feel more informed and empowered during labor.

8. How will my birth plan be considered during labor and delivery?

If you have specific preferences for your labor and delivery experience, such as natural birth methods, pain relief options, or who will be present in the delivery room, it's important to communicate these preferences with your doctor. While it's essential to remain flexible in case of unforeseen complications, having a clear discussion about your birth plan ensures that your doctor understands your wishes and can make every effort to accommodate them while prioritizing the health and safety of you and your baby.

9. What should I know about postpartum care and recovery?

The postpartum period is often overlooked in discussions about pregnancy and childbirth, but it's a critical time for both physical and emotional recovery. Ask your doctor what to expect in terms of postpartum care, including pain management, monitoring for complications like infections or blood clots, and breastfeeding support. It's also important to address the possibility of postpartum depression or anxiety and discuss available resources and support if you need help during your recovery.

10. How can I advocate for myself during pregnancy and labor?

Lastly, it's essential to feel empowered to ask questions, express concerns, and advocate for yourself throughout your pregnancy and childbirth journey. Don't hesitate to ask your doctor how you can best communicate your needs and preferences during labor and delivery, and how to ensure that your voice is heard in the decision-making process. Your healthcare provider should be a partner in your care, and open, respectful communication is key to making informed choices about your health and your baby's well-being.

In conclusion, navigating the myths and misconceptions about medical interventions during pregnancy can be challenging, but open and informed discussions with your healthcare provider can provide the clarity and confidence you need. By addressing myths such as the idea that C-sections are the "easy way out," that all pregnancies are the same, or that all medications should be avoided, women can better understand the reality of pregnancy and make informed decisions about their care. Additionally, knowing what questions to ask your doctor ensures that you are fully informed about the medical interventions that may be necessary and can advocate for yourself and your baby throughout the pregnancy and childbirth process.

Misconceptions About Labor and Delivery

L abor and delivery are often surrounded by a myriad of myths and misconceptions that can create confusion, anxiety, and unrealistic expectations for expectant mothers. From the belief that labor will begin right on the due date to the idea that walking can induce labor, these misconceptions can cause unnecessary stress as the mother-to-be approaches the end of her pregnancy. Furthermore, concerns about medical interventions, such as the use of epidurals, add another layer of complexity to the decisions that need to be made as the labor process begins. This chapter will address common myths about labor and delivery, clarify the truths behind these misconceptions, and provide a clear picture of what to expect in the delivery room.

Myth 16: Labor Starts on Your Due Date

One of the most persistent myths surrounding labor is the idea that it will begin precisely on the baby's due date. Many women circle the date on their calendar, eagerly anticipating the arrival of their child on that specific day. However, this myth is not based on medical reality, and the expectation that labor will begin on the due date can lead to unnecessary anxiety and disappointment when it doesn't happen.

The reality is that a due date is merely an estimate of when the baby is likely to be born, not a guaranteed timeline. A full-term pregnancy is considered to be anywhere from 37 to 42 weeks, and only about 5% of babies are actually born on their due date. The due date is typically calculated based on the first day of the woman's last menstrual period (LMP) or through early ultrasound measurements, but there are several factors that can influence the accuracy of this estimate, such as the length of the woman's menstrual cycle or the date of ovulation.

In truth, labor can start anytime within the full-term window, and many first-time mothers, in particular, tend to go into labor after their due date. Going past the due date is not uncommon, and in many cases, doctors will allow pregnancy to continue until 41 or even 42 weeks before considering interventions such as labor induction. However, if a pregnancy extends beyond 41 weeks, healthcare providers may monitor the baby more closely to ensure that the placenta is still functioning properly and that the baby is not experiencing any distress.

It is important for expectant mothers to understand that going past the due date does not necessarily indicate a problem. As long as the baby is healthy and there are no complications, many healthcare providers will recommend a "wait and see" approach, allowing labor to begin naturally. In some cases, a doctor may suggest certain measures to encourage labor to start, but the decision to induce labor is usually based on medical necessity rather than the mere passing of the due date.

By understanding that the due date is only an estimate and that labor can start anytime within the range of 37 to 42 weeks, expectant mothers can reduce their anxiety and better manage their expectations. Rather than focusing on the exact date, it is more helpful to think of the due date as a general timeframe and to prepare for labor to begin when the baby is ready.

Myth 17: Walking Induces Labor

Another common myth about labor is the idea that walking or engaging in other forms of physical activity can help induce labor. Many women, particularly those who are past their due date, are advised by well-meaning friends and family members to go for long walks, climb stairs, or perform squats in an effort to "kick start" labor. While it's true that exercise is generally beneficial for pregnant women and can help maintain physical fitness, there is little scientific evidence to support the notion that walking or other physical activities will induce labor.

The belief that walking can induce labor may stem from the idea that gravity will help the baby move down into the pelvis, which is an important part of the labor process. However, while walking may help the baby engage more deeply in the pelvis, it does not trigger the hormonal changes necessary to start labor. Labor is a complex process that involves the release of specific hormones, including oxytocin, which cause the uterus to contract and the cervix to dilate. These hormonal changes are regulated by both the mother's body and the baby, and they occur when the baby is ready to be born—not simply because of physical activity.

That said, walking can still be beneficial during late pregnancy and early labor. Physical activity, such as walking, can help improve circulation, relieve back pain, and reduce stress, all of which are helpful for overall well-being during pregnancy. Additionally, walking during early labor may help women cope with contractions and encourage the baby to move into an optimal position for birth. However, it is important to recognize that walking will not "bring on" labor if the body is not ready, and women should not overexert themselves in an attempt to speed up the process.

For women who are eager to meet their baby and are considering natural methods to induce labor, it is always best to consult with a healthcare provider before trying any interventions. While walking and staying active can be part of a healthy pregnancy routine, the onset of labor is ultimately controlled by physiological factors that cannot be forced by physical activity alone. In the meantime, women can focus on staying comfortable, relaxed, and prepared for labor to begin when the time is right.

Myth 18: Epidurals Can Harm the Baby

Epidural anesthesia is one of the most common forms of pain relief used during labor and delivery, but it is also the subject of numerous myths and misconceptions. One of the most persistent myths is the belief that epidurals can harm the baby, either by affecting the baby's development or by causing complications during birth. This myth can create unnecessary fear and guilt for women who are considering an epidural for pain management.

In reality, epidurals are considered a safe and effective form of pain relief for most women during labor, and there is no evidence to suggest that they cause harm to the baby. Epidurals work by delivering a combination of anesthetic and pain-relieving medications through a catheter placed in the lower back, which numbs the lower half of the body while allowing the woman to remain awake and alert. The medications used in an epidural are carefully controlled, and only a small amount crosses the placenta to reach the baby.

Studies have shown that babies born to mothers who receive epidurals do not experience any long-term developmental issues as a result of the anesthesia. In fact, the use of an epidural can help reduce maternal stress and exhaustion during labor, which can have a positive impact on both the mother and the baby. By allowing the mother to rest and manage her pain more effectively, an epidural can contribute to a more positive birth experience and reduce the risk of complications such as high blood pressure or prolonged labor.

However, like any medical intervention, epidurals do carry some potential risks and side effects. One of the most common side effects is a drop in the mother's blood pressure, which can reduce blood flow to the baby. To prevent this, healthcare providers typically administer fluids through an IV before the epidural is placed and closely monitor the mother's blood pressure throughout labor. In some cases, an epidural may cause the mother to experience temporary difficulty pushing, which can slightly prolong the second stage of labor. If this occurs, healthcare providers may assist with the delivery using forceps or a vacuum extractor.

It is also important to note that not all women are good candidates for epidural anesthesia. Women with certain medical conditions, such as low platelet counts or infections near the site where the epidural would be placed, may be advised against having an epidural. Additionally, some women may experience side effects such as a headache or temporary back pain after the epidural is administered.

Despite these potential risks, the overall safety profile of epidurals is well-established, and most women who choose to receive an epidural during labor report a positive experience. The decision to have an epidural is a personal one, and women should feel empowered to make the choice that is best for them based on their pain tolerance, birth plan, and medical advice from their healthcare provider.

The Truth Behind Labor and What to Expect in the Delivery Room

Understanding the truth about labor and delivery, as well as knowing what to expect in the delivery room, can help women feel more prepared and less anxious as they approach the birth of their child. While every labor experience is unique, there are some common truths about the process that can provide valuable insights for expectant mothers.

Labor typically unfolds in three stages: the first stage (early and active labor), the second stage (pushing and delivery of the baby), and the third stage (delivery of the placenta). The first stage of labor is often the longest and involves the gradual dilation and effacement (thinning) of the cervix as the body prepares for delivery. During this stage, contractions become more regular, frequent, and intense, signaling that labor is progressing.

Early labor, the initial phase of the first stage, can last for several hours or even days in some cases. During early labor, contractions are usually mild to moderate and may feel like menstrual cramps. Many women are able to stay at home during this phase, using comfort measures such as walking, taking warm baths, or practicing breathing techniques to cope with the discomfort.

As labor progresses into the active phase, contractions become more intense and frequent, and the cervix dilates more rapidly. This is often the point at which women are advised to go to the hospital or birthing center if they are not already there. During active labor, pain management options such as epidurals, nitrous oxide, or other medications may be offered, depending on the woman's preferences and the policies of the healthcare facility.

The second stage of labor begins when the cervix is fully dilated (10 centimeters) and the baby is ready to be pushed through the birth canal. This stage can last anywhere from a few minutes to a few hours, depending on factors such as the baby's position and the mother's ability to push effectively. During this stage, women may be guided by their healthcare provider to push during contractions, and they may be encouraged to change positions to facilitate the baby's descent through the birth canal. Many women find this stage to be physically intense but also empowering, as they actively work to bring their baby into the world. The healthcare team will closely monitor both the mother and baby during this time to ensure that labor is progressing safely.

Once the baby's head crowns (becomes visible), the healthcare provider may provide guidance on controlled pushing to prevent perineal tears or minimize the need for an episiotomy (a surgical incision to enlarge the vaginal opening). In some cases, the provider may assist with tools such as forceps or a vacuum extractor if the baby is having difficulty descending.

After the baby is born, the focus shifts to the third stage of labor—the delivery of the placenta. This stage typically occurs within 5 to 30 minutes after the baby is born and is much less physically demanding than the previous stages. The uterus will continue to contract, helping to detach and expel the placenta. Once the placenta is delivered, the healthcare team will inspect it to ensure that it is complete, as any remaining fragments in the uterus can cause complications such as infection or excessive bleeding.

Following the delivery of the placenta, the healthcare team will focus on monitoring the mother for signs of postpartum hemorrhage and ensuring that any necessary repairs, such as stitches for a tear or episiotomy, are completed. The mother and baby will typically have immediate skin-to-skin contact, which is encouraged for its many benefits, including promoting bonding, regulating the baby's body temperature, and initiating breastfeeding.

The Role of Medical Interventions in the Delivery Room

While many women hope for a natural or intervention-free birth, it's important to understand that medical interventions are sometimes necessary to ensure the safety of both the mother and baby. The key is to remain flexible and informed about the potential interventions that may arise during labor and delivery. Knowing what to expect can help women feel more prepared and empowered to make decisions if the situation calls for it.

Common medical interventions during labor include the use of intravenous (IV) fluids, continuous fetal monitoring, labor augmentation (such as with Pitocin), and pain relief options like epidurals. Each of these interventions has specific purposes, and while they may not always be part of a woman's original birth plan, they are often used to address medical concerns or to help labor progress more smoothly.

IV Fluids are commonly administered to women in labor to prevent dehydration and to ensure that medications (such as pain relief or antibiotics) can be delivered if needed. While IV fluids are a routine part of many hospital births, some women opt for intermittent monitoring or choose to stay mobile during labor by using wireless monitoring devices, depending on hospital policies.

Fetal Monitoring is used to track the baby's heart rate during labor, helping healthcare providers identify any signs of distress. Continuous electronic fetal monitoring involves placing sensors on the mother's abdomen to monitor the baby's heart rate and the frequency of contractions. Intermittent monitoring, on the other hand, may be used in low-risk pregnancies and involves periodic checks of the baby's heart rate using a handheld Doppler device. Continuous monitoring may be recommended for women with high-risk pregnancies, those who receive epidurals, or when labor is induced with medications like Pitocin.

Labor Induction and Augmentation: In some cases, labor needs to be induced or augmented (sped up) if it is not progressing naturally or if there are medical concerns. Induction is commonly done using medications such as Pitocin (a synthetic form of oxytocin) to stimulate contractions. Labor may also be induced by manually breaking the amniotic sac (a procedure known as amniotomy). Augmentation may be recommended if labor stalls or is progressing very slowly. While induction and augmentation can help labor progress more efficiently, they can also increase the intensity of contractions, which is why women may choose to use pain relief options like epidurals in conjunction with these interventions.

Pain Management: The choice of pain relief during labor is highly personal, and women have a range of options depending on their preferences and the circumstances of their labor. In addition to epidurals, other forms of pain management include intravenous pain medications, nitrous oxide (laughing gas), and natural methods such as breathing techniques, hydrotherapy (using water to ease pain), and massage. Each method has its own benefits and potential side effects, and it is essential for women to discuss their options with their healthcare provider in advance of labor so that they can make informed decisions based on their needs and preferences.

What to Expect Emotionally and Physically in the Delivery Room

The experience of labor and delivery can be both physically and emotionally overwhelming. For many women, the anticipation and excitement of meeting their baby are mixed with feelings of anxiety, pain, and uncertainty about what to expect. It's important to acknowledge that labor is an intense physical process, and every woman's experience will be different. However, understanding the key stages of labor and the potential interventions that may occur can help women feel more prepared.

Emotionally, many women experience a wide range of feelings throughout labor—from excitement and joy to frustration or fear, especially if labor doesn't go as planned. It's normal to feel a sense of loss of control at certain points during labor, particularly during intense contractions or when medical interventions become necessary. Having a supportive birth team, which may include a partner, doula, or family members, can provide emotional reassurance and help women stay focused on the process.

Physically, labor involves periods of intense contractions that become stronger and more frequent as labor progresses. Many women describe contractions as painful, but there are a variety of techniques that can help manage discomfort, including changing positions, using a birthing ball, practicing breathing exercises, or receiving pain relief through medication. The pushing phase requires focused effort, but the reward of seeing and holding the baby for the first time can be a powerful and trans-formative experience.

After the baby is born, the emotions of childbirth can be overwhelming, and many women describe feeling an immediate rush of love and relief when they hold their newborn. Others may experience more complex emotions, especially if the birth didn't go as planned or if they are recovering from a difficult labor. It's important to give yourself time to process these emotions and to reach out for support if needed.

Physically, the postpartum recovery process begins immediately after delivery.

The uterus will continue to contract to expel the placenta, and women may experience cramping or discomfort as their body begins to return to its pre-pregnancy state. The healthcare team will monitor the mother for signs of excessive bleeding or other complications, and they will provide care for any tears or stitches that may be required. The postpartum period is a time of healing and adjustment, and while it can be physically challenging, it is also a time of bonding with the baby and beginning the journey of parenthood.

Conclusion: Embracing the Reality of Labor and Delivery

The myths and misconceptions surrounding labor and delivery can create unrealistic expectations for many women. From the idea that labor will begin right on the due date to the belief that walking can induce labor, these myths can add unnecessary stress to an already emotional experience. Additionally, fears about medical interventions, such as the use of epidurals, can cause anxiety and uncertainty for women as they prepare for childbirth.

By understanding the truths behind these myths and gaining a clearer picture of what to expect in the delivery room, women can approach labor and delivery with greater confidence and knowledge. Every labor experience is unique, and while some aspects of labor are unpredictable, being informed about the stages of labor, pain management options, and potential interventions can help women make empowered decisions for themselves and their babies.

Ultimately, the goal of labor and delivery is a healthy outcome for both mother and baby. Whether labor unfolds naturally or with the help of medical interventions, the process of bringing a child into the world is a powerful and trans-formative experience. By letting go of myths and embracing the realities of labor, women can focus on the journey ahead and the incredible reward of meeting their new baby.

Postpartum Myths

The postpartum period, often referred to as the "fourth trimester," is a critical and trans-formative time for new mothers. It's a phase filled with physical recovery, emotional changes, and the new responsibilities of caring for a newborn. However, just as with pregnancy and childbirth, the postpartum experience is surrounded by numerous myths and misconceptions that can lead to unrealistic expectations, guilt, or confusion. From the belief that breastfeeding comes naturally to everyone, to the pressure to quickly regain one's pre-pregnancy body, these myths can overshadow the complexities of postpartum recovery and adjustment. In this chapter, we will explore three pervasive postpartum myths—breastfeeding, body recovery, and postpartum depression—and uncover the realities of this unique stage of motherhood.

Myth 19: Breastfeeding is Easy for Everyone

One of the most common misconceptions about the postpartum period is the belief that breastfeeding is natural and easy for all mothers. Many women, especially first-time mothers, expect that breastfeeding will come naturally and smoothly as soon as their baby is born. This assumption is often reinforced by images in the media, which portray breastfeeding as an effortless, serene bonding experience between mother and baby. While breastfeeding is indeed a natural biological process, it is not always easy, and many women face challenges that can make the experience far more difficult than anticipated.

In reality, breastfeeding can be a complex and sometimes painful process that requires patience, practice, and support. Common difficulties include issues with latch, low milk supply, nipple pain or damage, engorgement, and infections like mastitis. Some babies may have difficulty breastfeeding due to tongue-tie, jaundice, or other medical issues, while some mothers may struggle with their milk production, often worrying that they're not providing enough nourishment for their baby.

Latch problems, in particular, are one of the most frequently encountered challenges for new mothers. A good latch is essential for efficient milk transfer and to prevent nipple pain or damage, but achieving a proper latch can take time. Many mothers experience cracked or sore nipples in the early days of breastfeeding, which can make the process incredibly painful and frustrating. Additionally, a baby's feeding schedule can be unpredictable and exhausting, especially during the first few weeks, when babies often feed frequently and irregularly. This constant demand can leave new mothers feeling overwhelmed, sleep-deprived, and uncertain about whether they're doing it "right."

Low milk supply is another common concern, although it is often misdiagnosed. Many women worry that their baby isn't getting enough milk, particularly when the baby seems to want to nurse frequently. However, frequent feeding is normal for newborns, and it is not necessarily a sign of low supply. In most cases, the body will produce enough milk as long as the baby is nursing regularly and effectively. However, there are situations where genuine supply issues can arise, such as hormonal imbalances, previous breast surgery, or medical conditions that affect milk production. In these cases, seeking help from a lactation consultant or healthcare provider is crucial to determine the cause and find solutions.

The myth that breastfeeding is easy for everyone can also create feelings of inadequacy or guilt in mothers who struggle with it. Women who find breastfeeding painful, stressful, or unsustainable may feel as though they are failing as mothers if they choose to supplement with formula or switch to formula feeding entirely. This pressure can be exacerbated by societal messages that emphasize breastfeeding as the best and only way to bond with a baby or provide adequate nutrition. While breastfeeding has well-documented health benefits for both mother and baby, it is important to recognize that not all mothers are able to breastfeed, and that formula feeding can also support a healthy, thriving baby.

Support is key to overcoming breastfeeding challenges, and it is essential for mothers to have access to resources such as lactation consultants, breastfeeding support groups, and knowledgeable healthcare providers. These resources can provide guidance on latch techniques, supply issues, and other concerns, helping to ease the difficulties that many new mothers face. For those who are unable to breastfeed or choose not to, it is important to remember that there are many ways to bond with and nourish a baby, and that a mother's worth is not defined by her ability to breastfeed.

Myth 20: You'll Bounce Back to Your Pre-Pregnancy Body Quickly

The pressure to "bounce back" to one's pre-pregnancy body immediately after giving birth is another widespread postpartum myth. This myth is perpetuated by images of celebrities or influencers who appear to regain their pre-baby figures within weeks of giving birth, often highlighting flat stomachs and toned bodies as if pregnancy never happened. For many women, this creates unrealistic expectations about their own postpartum recovery and body image, leading to frustration, self-doubt, and even feelings of failure when their bodies don't "bounce back" as quickly as expected.

In reality, the postpartum body is recovering from one of the most physically demanding experiences a woman can undergo: pregnancy and childbirth. During pregnancy, the body undergoes significant changes, including weight gain, changes in muscle tone, and the stretching of the abdominal muscles. After delivery, it takes time for the uterus to shrink back to its normal size, for the abdominal muscles to heal, and for the body to shed the extra fluid and fat that accumulated during pregnancy.

For most women, it is normal to retain some extra weight after giving birth, and it can take months or even longer to return to their pre-pregnancy weight and fitness level. The rate at which a woman's body recovers varies depending on several factors, including genetics, pre-pregnancy fitness, the type of birth she had (vaginal or C-section), and whether she is breastfeeding. Breastfeeding can help with postpartum weight loss because it burns extra calories, but it also increases hunger, which may lead some women to consume more food to maintain their energy levels.

It's also important to recognize that for some women, their bodies may never fully return to their pre-pregnancy state—and that's perfectly normal. Stretch marks, changes in breast size, and looser skin are common after pregnancy, and they are a testament to the incredible work the body has done in creating and nurturing new life. However, societal pressures often push women to view these changes as flaws, leading to feelings of dissatisfaction with their postpartum bodies.

The myth of the "bounce back" culture can also drive women to engage in unhealthy behaviors, such as crash dieting or intense exercise routines, too soon after giving birth. The postpartum period is a time of healing and recovery, and it's crucial for new mothers to prioritize rest, nutrition, and gentle physical activity that supports their body's healing process. Rushing into restrictive diets or vigorous workouts can put unnecessary strain on a body that is still recovering from childbirth and may increase the risk of injury or complications.

It's essential for women to give themselves grace during the postpartum period and to understand that their bodies have undergone a profound transformation. Rather than focusing on the idea of "bouncing back," it's more helpful to think of postpartum recovery as a gradual process of healing, rebuilding strength, and adjusting to the new demands of motherhood. The goal should be to feel healthy, strong, and confident in one's body, rather than striving to meet unrealistic expectations of physical appearance.

Myth 21: Postpartum Depression is Just "Baby Blues"

Postpartum depression (PPD) is often misunderstood and minimized as simply an extension of the "baby blues." While it is true that many new mothers experience mood swings, irritability, and feelings of sadness or overwhelm in the days or weeks following childbirth, these symptoms typically subside within a couple of weeks. This temporary mood disturbance, known as the baby blues, is thought to be related to the rapid hormonal changes that occur after delivery, combined with the physical exhaustion and emotional adjustment of caring for a newborn.

Postpartum depression, however, is a more serious and long-lasting condition that affects approximately 10-15% of women after childbirth. Unlike the baby blues, which tend to resolve on their own, postpartum depression can persist for months if left untreated and can significantly impact a woman's ability to function and care for her baby. The symptoms of PPD are more severe and may include intense feelings of sadness, hopelessness, or worthlessness, difficulty bonding with the baby, withdrawal from family and friends, extreme fatigue or insomnia, and, in some cases, thoughts of self-harm or harm to the baby.

The myth that postpartum depression is merely an exaggerated version of the baby blues can prevent women from seeking the help they need. Many women feel ashamed or embarrassed about their symptoms, fearing that they are failing as mothers or that they should be able to "snap out of it." This stigma surrounding PPD can lead to a delay in diagnosis and treatment, prolonging the suffering of both the mother and her family.

It is essential to recognize that postpartum depression is a medical condition, not a personal failing, and it is treatable. The exact cause of PPD is not fully understood, but it is believed to be related to a combination of hormonal changes, genetic predisposition, and environmental factors. Women who have a history of depression or anxiety, a lack of social support, or who experience a traumatic birth are at higher risk for developing postpartum depression.

Treatment for PPD often includes therapy, medication, or a combination of both. Cognitive-behavioral therapy (CBT) and other forms of counseling can help women manage their symptoms, process their emotions, and develop coping strategies. In some cases, antidepressant medications may be prescribed to help regulate mood, and these medications are often considered safe for breastfeeding mothers.

It is also important for partners, family members, and friends to be aware of the signs of postpartum depression and to offer support without judgment. Encouraging new mothers to seek help and providing practical assistance with childcare, household tasks, or simply offering a listening ear can make a significant difference in a woman's recovery from PPD.

Understanding the Realities of the Postpartum Experience

The postpartum period is a time of profound change, both physically and emotionally. In addition to the specific challenges outlined above, The postpartum period is a time of profound change, both physically and emotionally. In addition to the specific challenges outlined above, new mothers are often navigating the complexities of their own recovery while adjusting to the demands of caring for a newborn. The realities of this period can vary widely from person to person, depending on factors like health, support systems, and the temperament of the baby, but the common experience is one of transition and adjustment.

Physical Recovery After Childbirth

Physically, the body undergoes a significant recovery process after childbirth, regardless of whether the birth was vaginal or via cesarean section. Many women experience soreness, fatigue, and discomfort for several weeks as their bodies heal. For those who have had vaginal births, recovering from tearing or an episiotomy may involve managing perineal pain and swelling, while women who had C-sections will need to care for their incision site and manage the discomfort associated with major abdominal surgery.

In addition to these immediate physical recovery needs, there are also postpartum changes that can take some time to resolve. For example, lochia, a vaginal discharge that occurs as the uterus sheds its lining, typically continues for several weeks. Hormonal fluctuations can also cause night sweats, mood swings, and changes in appetite. All of this can be overwhelming, especially when coupled with the sleeplessness that comes with caring for a newborn.

Breastfeeding mothers may also experience additional physical challenges, including nipple pain, engorgement, or mastitis (a painful breast infection). Some women experience changes in breast size and shape after breastfeeding, and hormonal changes related to lactation can further impact mood and energy levels.

It's important for postpartum women to prioritize their own recovery during this time, seeking help when needed and allowing themselves the space to heal. This can mean asking for support from partners, family members, or friends, and making use of postpartum resources such as lactation consultants or pelvic floor physical therapists. Unfortunately, the myth that new mothers should "bounce back" quickly can make it harder for women to feel comfortable taking this time for themselves.

The Emotional Rollercoaster

Emotionally, the postpartum period can be just as intense, if not more so, than the physical recovery. For some women, this period is marked by feelings of joy, connection, and fulfillment as they bond with their baby. However, for many others, it is also a time of intense emotional challenges, including feelings of anxiety, overwhelm, sadness, or frustration. These feelings can be compounded by the exhaustion that comes with caring for a newborn, sleep deprivation, and the pressure to meet societal expectations around motherhood.

One of the most difficult realities for new mothers is the sense of isolation that can come during the postpartum period. While motherhood is often idealized in our culture, many new mothers find that the day-to-day realities of caring for a newborn are far more challenging than they had anticipated. The constant demands of feeding, soothing, and changing diapers can leave women feeling isolated from their pre-baby social lives, particularly if they don't have a strong support network or are struggling with the emotional toll of postpartum depression or anxiety.

It's crucial for mothers to recognize that they are not alone in these feelings and that asking for help is not a sign of weakness. Many women find solace in connecting with other new mothers through postpartum support groups or online communities. Additionally, mental health professionals who specialize in postpartum issues can provide valuable guidance and support during this transitional period.

The Importance of Support Systems

A strong support system is one of the most important factors in helping new mothers navigate the postpartum period. Partners, family members, and friends can play a key role in providing emotional support, helping with household tasks, and giving the new mother time to rest and recover. The "it takes a village" adage rings particularly true when it comes to postpartum recovery.

Partners, in particular, have a vital role in supporting the emotional and physical well-being of the new mother. Taking on responsibilities such as diaper changes, nighttime feedings (if bottle feeding is possible), and providing emotional support can make a significant difference in how a mother copes during this period. Open communication between partners about needs, expectations, and feelings is crucial to maintaining a healthy relationship during this challenging time.

Additionally, new mothers should not hesitate to reach out to healthcare professionals if they experience any physical or emotional complications after childbirth. Whether it's persistent pain, trouble breastfeeding, or feelings of anxiety or depression, it's important to address these issues early to ensure proper treatment and support.

Postpartum Expectations vs. Reality

It's important to acknowledge that the postpartum period may not look like what many women expect. From social media posts to celebrity narratives, there is often an idealized image of new motherhood that doesn't reflect the realities most women face. This can create feelings of inadequacy or self-doubt for mothers whose experiences don't align with these images.

In truth, the postpartum period is a deeply personal and variable experience. For some, it may be a time filled with joy and bonding, while for others, it may be marked by physical discomfort, emotional upheaval, and fatigue. There is no right or wrong way to experience this time, and each mother's journey is unique.

Being realistic about what to expect can help mothers feel more prepared for the challenges of the postpartum period. Recognizing that recovery takes time, that breastfeeding may not be easy, and that emotional struggles like postpartum depression are real and treatable can alleviate some of the pressure that new mothers often feel.

Conclusion

Understanding the myths and realities of the postpartum experience is essential for helping new mothers navigate this complex and challenging time. By dispelling myths such as the ease of breastfeeding, the expectation of quickly returning to a pre-pregnancy body, and the misconception that postpartum depression is just the baby blues, women can approach the postpartum period with a more realistic and compassionate mindset.

The postpartum journey is not one-size-fits-all, and every mother's experience will be different. By focusing on healing, seeking support, and being gentle with themselves, new mothers can find their way through this transformative period with the understanding that they are not alone and that their experiences—whether filled with joy or challenges—are valid and important.

Cultural and Societal Myths About Pregnancy

Pregnancy is a universal experience, yet it is shaped by the cultural, societal, and individual contexts in which it occurs. Around the world, different cultures and societies have their own beliefs, traditions, and myths surrounding pregnancy, many of which are passed down from generation to generation. While some of these beliefs are rooted in wisdom or historical practices, others are based on misconceptions that can create unnecessary anxiety or unrealistic expectations for expectant mothers. In this chapter, we explore some of the most pervasive cultural and societal myths about pregnancy, including those related to older mothers, the emotional expectations surrounding pregnancy, and the fear of recurrent miscarriage. We will also examine how culture influences pregnancy beliefs and why it is essential to address these myths with evidence-based information.

Myth 22: Older Mothers Can't Have Healthy Pregnancies

One of the most entrenched myths across many societies is the belief that older mothers—typically defined as women who are 35 or older—are unable to have healthy pregnancies or are at significantly higher risk of complications. This myth often comes with societal judgments that suggest women who wait until later in life to have children are selfish or irresponsible, prioritizing their careers or personal goals over motherhood. While it is true that maternal age can influence certain aspects of pregnancy and fertility, the assumption that older mothers cannot have healthy pregnancies is both outdated and misleading.

In reality, many women over 35 go on to have healthy pregnancies and deliver healthy babies. Advances in medical care, prenatal testing, and fertility treatments have made it possible for women in their late 30s, 40s, and even beyond to conceive and carry pregnancies safely. While it is true that fertility declines with age, and the risk of certain complications, such as gestational diabetes, preeclampsia, and chromosomal abnormalities, may be higher for older mothers, the vast majority of women in this age group still experience successful pregnancies.

One of the key concerns for older mothers is the increased risk of chromosomal abnormalities, such as Down syndrome, which becomes more prevalent as a woman's eggs age. However, it is important to note that while the risk increases, the overall likelihood of a baby being born with such a condition remains relatively low. For example, at age 35, the risk of having a baby with Down syndrome is about 1 in 350, and by age 40, it increases to about 1 in 100. Prenatal testing, such as non-invasive prenatal testing (NIPT), amniocentesis, and chorionic villus sampling (CVS), can provide parents with accurate information about the health of their baby, allowing them to make informed decisions about their pregnancy.

In addition to concerns about genetic conditions, older mothers may also face a higher likelihood of complications during pregnancy, such as high blood pressure or gestational diabetes. However, these risks can often be managed with appropriate medical care and lifestyle modifications. Regular prenatal checkups, healthy eating, staying active, and following medical advice can go a long way in mitigating these risks and ensuring a healthy pregnancy for older mothers.

It is also important to acknowledge the benefits of having children later in life.

Many older mothers are in a stable financial and emotional position, having established their careers and personal lives before deciding to start a family. This stability can contribute to a more positive pregnancy and parenting experience, as older mothers may feel more prepared for the challenges of motherhood. Additionally, studies have shown that older mothers tend to have better emotional well-being during pregnancy and are more likely to seek and follow medical advice, which can contribute to better outcomes for both mother and baby.

While it is essential to recognize that age can be a factor in pregnancy, the idea that older mothers are inherently at risk or irresponsible for choosing to have children later in life is a harmful myth. With proper medical care, older mothers can and do have healthy pregnancies, and the decision to become a parent should be respected, regardless of a woman's age.

Myth 23: Pregnancy is a Time of Joy for Everyone

The cultural narrative surrounding pregnancy often paints it as a time of pure joy and excitement, with expectant mothers glowing with happiness as they prepare to welcome a new life into the world. This idealized view of pregnancy can create a false expectation that all women should feel joyful and fulfilled during this time, and that any negative emotions or struggles are abnormal or a sign of failure. However, the reality is that pregnancy is a complex emotional experience, and not all women feel joy or excitement throughout the entire process. For some, pregnancy can be marked by feelings of anxiety, depression, fear, or even ambivalence.

There are many reasons why a woman might not feel joyful during pregnancy, and these reasons are deeply personal and varied. Some women may struggle with the physical discomforts of pregnancy, such as morning sickness, fatigue, or pain, which can make it difficult to feel positive about the experience. Others may have concerns about the health of their baby, financial stability, or the impact of becoming a parent on their personal and professional lives.

Additionally, women who have experienced previous pregnancy loss or infertility may find it challenging to fully embrace the joy of pregnancy due to lingering fears of loss or disappointment.

Mental health conditions, such as prenatal depression or anxiety, can also significantly impact a woman's emotional experience during pregnancy. Despite the common belief that depression and anxiety only occur postpartum, many women experience these conditions during pregnancy, often referred to as antenatal or prenatal depression. This can manifest as feelings of sadness, hopelessness, irritability, or overwhelming worry, and it is essential for women to seek support if they are struggling with their mental health during pregnancy.

The myth that pregnancy is a universally joyful experience can prevent women from acknowledging their true feelings and seeking help when needed. Many women feel ashamed or guilty for not feeling the way they think they "should," and this can lead to isolation or a reluctance to speak openly about their struggles. It is important to create a more nuanced and compassionate narrative around pregnancy that recognizes the full range of emotions that women may experience, from joy and excitement to fear and uncertainty.

Support from healthcare providers, partners, family, and friends is crucial in helping women navigate the emotional challenges of pregnancy. Prenatal mental health services, counseling, and support groups can provide valuable resources for women who are struggling with their emotions during pregnancy. By normalizing the reality that pregnancy is not always a time of unmitigated joy, we can create a more supportive and understanding environment for expectant mothers.

Myth 24: If You've Had a Miscarriage, You're Likely to Have Another

Miscarriage is one of the most difficult experiences a woman can go through, and the emotional toll can be overwhelming. Unfortunately, there are many myths and misconceptions about miscarriage that can exacerbate the pain and anxiety of those who have experienced it. One of the most common myths is the belief that if a woman has had a miscarriage, she is likely to have another one. This myth can create fear and anxiety for women who are trying to conceive again after a loss, leading them to believe that their bodies are somehow "broken" or that they are destined to experience repeated miscarriages.

The truth is that most women who experience a miscarriage go on to have healthy pregnancies and deliver healthy babies. According to the American College of Obstetricians and Gynecologists (ACOG), approximately 10-20% of known pregnancies end in miscarriage, with the actual number likely higher due to early losses that occur before a woman realizes she is pregnant. The vast majority of miscarriages are caused by chromosomal abnormalities in the embryo, which occur by chance and are not likely to repeat in subsequent pregnancies.

For women who have had one miscarriage, the risk of having another is only slightly higher than the general population. Studies have shown that after one miscarriage, the likelihood of a successful subsequent pregnancy is around 85%. Even for women who have had two or more miscarriages, the chance of having a healthy pregnancy is still high. However, women who have experienced multiple miscarriages (recurrent pregnancy loss) may benefit from further medical evaluation to identify any underlying factors that could be contributing to the losses, such as hormonal imbalances, uterine abnormalities, or autoimmune conditions.

The myth that miscarriage is likely to recur can create significant emotional distress for women who are trying to conceive after a loss. Many women experience heightened anxiety during their subsequent pregnancies, particularly in the early weeks, as they fear another miscarriage. This anxiety can be compounded by societal attitudes that often discourage open discussions about miscarriage, leaving women to cope with their fears and grief in isolation.

It is essential to provide women who have experienced miscarriage with accurate information and emotional support. Counseling and support groups can offer a safe space for women to process their grief and fears, while medical providers can offer reassurance and guidance for future pregnancies. By dispelling the myth that miscarriage is likely to happen again, we can help women move forward with hope and confidence in their ability to have a healthy pregnancy.

The Influence of Culture on Pregnancy Beliefs

Cultural beliefs and traditions play a significant role in shaping how women experience pregnancy. Around the world, different cultures have their own practices, taboos, and myths related to pregnancy, many of which are passed down through generations. While some of these cultural beliefs can provide comfort and guidance, others may perpetuate harmful misconceptions that contribute to fear, anxiety, or even dangerous practices.

For example, in some cultures, certain foods or activities are believed to influence the outcome of a pregnancy, such as the gender of the baby or the health of the mother and child. While these beliefs may be deeply ingrained in cultural traditions, they are often based on superstition rather than scientific evidence. In other cases, cultural taboos surrounding pregnancy can lead to harmful practices, such as restricting a woman's access to certain types of medical care or discouraging her from seeking help for mental health concerns.

At the same time, cultural beliefs can also offer valuable support and connection during pregnancy. Many cultures have rituals and practices that celebrate pregnancy and honor the role of mothers, providing a sense of community and belonging during this trans-formative time. For example, in some cultures, there are special ceremonies or gatherings to bless the mother and baby, provide gifts, or share wisdom from older generations. These practices can create a sense of support and solidarity, reminding women that they are part of a long lineage of motherhood.

However, it is essential to balance cultural traditions with modern medical understanding. While some cultural beliefs may be comforting, others may conflict with evidence-based practices that prioritize maternal and fetal health. For example, in some cultures, women are discouraged from seeking prenatal care or using certain medical interventions due to traditional beliefs or taboos. In such cases, it's crucial to promote a dialogue that respects cultural values while also encouraging the use of safe, modern healthcare practices.

Healthcare providers must be culturally sensitive when working with expectant mothers from diverse backgrounds. This includes understanding the cultural beliefs that may influence a woman's pregnancy experience and addressing any myths or misconceptions with empathy and respect. By doing so, healthcare providers can build trust with their patients and provide the best possible care that aligns with both cultural values and medical science.

In some instances, cultural and societal myths about pregnancy can be particularly harmful. For example, in certain societies, there is a strong emphasis on producing male offspring, leading to pressure on pregnant women to conform to specific gender-related expectations. This can create anxiety and disappointment if the baby's sex does not align with cultural preferences, potentially affecting the woman's emotional well-being during pregnancy. Similarly, in some cultures, women may be blamed or stigmatized if they experience complications such as miscarriage or infertility, reinforcing feelings of shame or inadequacy.

Breaking down these harmful cultural myths requires a combination of education, community engagement, and support. It's important to create environments where women can speak openly about their experiences and concerns without fear of judgment or stigma. Education campaigns that address common myths and provide evidence-based information about pregnancy can help dispel misconceptions and empower women to make informed choices about their health and the health of their baby.

Furthermore, the role of family and community support cannot be under-stated. In many cultures, family members play a significant role in the pregnancy journey, offering advice, care, and support to the expectant mother. This network of support is invaluable, especially in cultures where extended family plays a central role in raising children. However, it is essential to ensure that this support is balanced with the mother's autonomy and access to accurate medical information. Families should be encouraged to provide emotional and practical support while also respecting the mother's choices and decisions regarding her pregnancy and childbirth.

In today's globalized world, many women navigate the intersection of traditional cultural beliefs and modern healthcare practices. This can create tension or confusion as they try to reconcile the advice of older family mem-bers or cultural traditions with the recommendations of healthcare providers. Open communication, education, and respect for diverse perspectives are key to helping women feel empowered to make the best decisions for themselves and their babies.

Cultural competency is increasingly recognized as a vital aspect of prenatal and maternal healthcare. Healthcare providers must be trained to understand and respect the diverse cultural beliefs and practices of the populations they serve. This includes being aware of how cultural myths may influence a woman's perception of pregnancy, her relationship with healthcare providers, and her willingness to seek medical care. By fostering an inclusive and respectful healthcare environment, providers can help ensure that all women receive the care they need, regardless of their cultural background.

In conclusion, cultural and societal beliefs about pregnancy are deeply ingrained in many traditions, but they must be carefully examined in light of modern medical knowledge. While some cultural practices provide valuable support and connection, others may perpetuate myths or misconceptions that can impact a woman's physical and emotional well-being. By addressing these myths with empathy and respect, and by promoting education and evidence-based healthcare, we can help women navigate the complexities of pregnancy in a way that honors both their cultural heritage and their health needs.

Debunking Myths About Twins and Multiple Pregnancies

Twins and multiple pregnancies have always fascinated people, and over time, a variety of myths and misconceptions have emerged about what causes twins, the risks associated with carrying more than one baby, and how multiple pregnancies differ from singleton pregnancies. Some of these myths are grounded in outdated beliefs, while others arise from misunderstandings about genetics, fertility, and medical advancements. In this chapter, we will explore common myths about twins and multiple pregnancies, debunk them using scientific evidence, and delve into the fascinating science behind how multiple pregnancies occur. Understanding the truth behind these myths can help expectant mothers, families, and society as a whole have a clearer perspective on what it means to carry twins or other multiples.

Myth 25: You Can Only Have Twins if It Runs in the Family

One of the most pervasive myths about twins is the belief that you can only have twins if they run in your family. While family history can play a role in increasing the likelihood of having certain types of twins, particularly fraternal twins, this is not a universal rule. The idea that twins are strictly the result of genetics is overly simplistic and ignores other factors that can influence the chances of having multiples.

There are two main types of twins: fraternal (dizygotic) and identical (monozygotic). Fraternal twins result from the fertilization of two separate eggs by two different sperm, while identical twins occur when a single fertilized egg splits into two embryos. The key distinction here is that fraternal twins are influenced by genetic factors, while identical twins happen by chance and are not influenced by family history.

Fraternal twins are more common than identical twins, and the likelihood of having fraternal twins can indeed be influenced by family history. If a woman's family has a history of fraternal twins, particularly on her maternal side, she may have a higher chance of releasing more than one egg during ovulation, increasing the likelihood of having fraternal twins. However, this genetic predisposition is not a guarantee that she will have twins, nor does it apply to all women equally.

Interestingly, the genetic predisposition for fraternal twins is thought to be passed down through the mother's side of the family. This is because it is the woman's ovulation process that determines whether more than one egg will be released during a menstrual cycle. Men can carry the gene for hyper ovulation and pass it on to their daughters, but their family history of twins does not directly increase their own chances of fathering twins, unless they partner with someone who carries the same trait.

In contrast, identical twins occur randomly and are not influenced by genetic factors. The splitting of a single fertilized egg into two embryos is a rare event that happens in about 3 to 4 per 1,000 births worldwide, regardless of the mother's age, ethnicity, or family history. This means that anyone can have identical twins, regardless of whether they run in the family.

Aside from genetics, other factors can increase the chances of having twins or multiples. One significant factor is the use of fertility treatments, such as in vitro fertilization (IVF) or medications that stimulate ovulation. These treatments can increase the likelihood of multiple eggs being released or implanted, leading to fraternal twins or even higher-order multiples (triplets, quadruplets, etc.). Additionally, maternal age plays a role: women over the age of 30, particularly those in their mid-1970s to early 40s, are more likely to release more than one egg during ovulation, which can result in fraternal twins.

In summary, while having fraternal twins may be more likely if it runs in your family, especially on the mother's side, identical twins are entirely random and unrelated to genetics. Moreover, factors like maternal age, fertility treatments, and other biological processes can increase the likelihood of having twins, even if there is no family history. Therefore, the idea that twins can only happen if they run in the family is not entirely accurate, and many people have twins without any family predisposition.

Myth 26: Twin Pregnancies Are Always Riskier

Another widespread myth is that twin pregnancies are inherently more dangerous or complicated than singleton pregnancies. While it is true that twin pregnancies come with some unique challenges and risks, the assumption that they are always high-risk or fraught with complications is misleading and can cause undue anxiety for expectant mothers carrying twins or multiples.

To understand why this myth persists, it is important to recognize that twin pregnancies do indeed have a higher likelihood of certain complications compared to singleton pregnancies. For example, women carrying twins are at an increased risk of preterm birth, low birth weight, gestational diabetes, preeclampsia, and cesarean delivery. These risks are largely related to the fact that carrying more than one baby places additional physical demands on the mother's body, and the babies themselves may compete for space and nutrients in the womb, which can affect their growth and development.

Preterm birth is one of the most common concerns in twin pregnancies.

Approximately 60% of twins are born before 37 weeks of gestation, compared to only about 10% of singletons. Because twins often have less time to fully develop in the womb, they are more likely to be born at a lower birth weight and may require additional medical care, such as time in the neonatal intensive care unit (NICU). However, with modern medical advancements, many premature babies, including twins, thrive with the appropriate care and support.

Gestational diabetes and preeclampsia are also more common in twin pregnancies due to the increased strain on the mother's body. Gestational diabetes occurs when the body cannot produce enough insulin to manage the increased demand for glucose during pregnancy, while preeclampsia is characterized by high blood pressure and damage to organs such as the liver and kidneys. Both conditions can pose risks to the mother and babies if left untreated, but with regular monitoring and medical care, these complications can often be managed effectively.

While these risks are real, it is essential to note that not all twin pregnancies result in complications, and many women go on to have healthy pregnancies and deliver healthy babies. The key to managing a twin pregnancy is receiving appropriate prenatal care and working closely with healthcare providers to monitor the mother's health and the development of the babies. Regular ultrasounds, monitoring for signs of preterm labor, and managing conditions like gestational diabetes can help ensure a safe pregnancy and delivery.

It is also worth mentioning that twin pregnancies vary depending on whether the twins are fraternal or identical, and whether they share a placenta or have their own. Identical twins who share a placenta (monochorionic twins) are at higher risk for complications such as twin-to-twin transfusion syndrome (TTTS), where one twin receives more blood flow than the other, potentially leading to growth disparities or health issues. However, this condition can often be detected early through routine ultrasounds and treated with specialized procedures if necessary.

Additionally, advances in obstetric care have improved outcomes for twin pregnancies over the years. Many of the complications associated with multiple pregnancies can be managed effectively with careful monitoring, early detection, and timely medical intervention. Women carrying twins are typically considered to have a higher-risk pregnancy, which means they will receive more frequent prenatal visits and ultrasounds to ensure both mother and babies are healthy. This increased level of care allows healthcare providers to address any potential issues before they become serious problems.

In short, while twin pregnancies do come with certain risks, they are not necessarily "dangerous" or doomed to complications. With proper medical care, most women carrying twins can have successful pregnancies and healthy babies. The idea that all twin pregnancies are inherently high-risk is a myth, and women should feel reassured that modern medicine provides the tools and knowledge needed to manage the unique aspects of multiple pregnancies.

The Science Behind Multiple Pregnancies

The occurrence of twins or multiples is a fascinating area of reproductive science, influenced by a combination of genetics, environmental factors, and medical advancements. Understanding the biology behind how multiple pregnancies happen can help dispel many of the myths surrounding twins and offer insight into the factors that increase the likelihood of having multiples.

As mentioned earlier, there are two main types of twins: fraternal (dizygotic) and identical (monozygotic). Fraternal twins occur when two separate eggs are released during ovulation and are fertilized by two different sperm. Because they come from two different eggs, fraternal twins are genetically no more similar than any other siblings—they share about 50% of their DNA. Fraternal twins can be of the same sex or different sexes, and they may look quite different from one another.

Fraternal twins are more common than identical twins and are influenced by several factors. One of the most significant factors is maternal age. Women over the age of 30, particularly those in their late 30s and early 40s, are more likely to release multiple eggs during ovulation, which increases the likelihood of fraternal twins. This is because, as a woman ages, her body may respond to declining fertility by releasing more than one egg in a single cycle.

The use of fertility treatments, such as ovulation-stimulating drugs or IVF, also significantly increases the chances of having fraternal twins. These treatments often involve stimulating the ovaries to produce multiple eggs, which can result in the fertilization of more than one egg and the development of twins or higher-order multiples.

Identical twins, on the other hand, occur when a single fertilized egg splits into two embryos. This splitting happens randomly and is not influenced by genetics or external factors. Identical twins share 100% of their DNA, which is why they look nearly identical and are always of the same sex. The exact cause of the egg's splitting is not fully understood, but it is thought to be a spontaneous event that occurs in about 3-4 per 1,000 births worldwide.

In addition to fraternal and identical twins, there are other types of multiples that occur, such as triplets, quadruplets, and even higher-order multiples, though these are far less common. Like fraternal twins, higher-order multiples typically result from the fertilization of multiple eggs, often due to fertility treatments or certain genetic predispositions. In some cases, a combination of both fraternal and identical twinning can occur, such as when one egg splits (resulting in identical twins) and another separate egg is fertilized (resulting in a fraternal triplet). These types of occurrences further showcase the complex nature of multiple pregnancies.

The science behind how multiple pregnancies occur is grounded in both biology and reproductive technology, but there are still some unknowns. For example, scientists are still researching the factors that cause a fertilized egg to split and result in identical twins. What is known is that there are certain populations and genetic traits that have higher incidences of fraternal twins. For example, women of African descent, particularly those from West Africa, have a higher incidence of fraternal twins compared to women of Asian descent, who have the lowest rates.

There are also other interesting scientific factors related to multiple pregnancies. For example, women who have had multiple pregnancies before (parity) or who are taller and heavier are more likely to conceive fraternal twins. It's theorized that taller women may have larger pelvic cavities and more nutrients available to support multiple pregnancies, while a higher body mass index (BMI) may influence hormone levels and ovulation patterns.

Another intriguing aspect of the science behind twins and multiples is the phenomenon of "vanishing twin syndrome." In some pregnancies, particularly those involving IVF, early ultrasounds may detect more than one embryo, but one of the embryos fails to develop or is absorbed into the body, resulting in a singleton pregnancy by the time of birth. This is not uncommon and may occur in up to 20-30% of twin pregnancies. While it can be distressing for parents who have initially expected twins, it's important to understand that this is a natural process, often happening very early in pregnancy.

Prenatal Care for Multiple Pregnancies

Prenatal care for twins and other multiples is often more intensive than for singleton pregnancies. Given the increased risk of complications, women carrying multiples typically have more frequent prenatal visits and ultrasounds to monitor the growth and development of the babies. The goal of this enhanced care is to detect and manage any potential issues as early as possible, helping to ensure the healthiest possible outcome for both the mother and the babies.

In many cases, women carrying twins or multiples are advised to gain more weight than those carrying singletons. This is because the nutritional demands of carrying more than one baby are greater, and adequate weight gain can support fetal growth. The recommended weight gain for a twin pregnancy is usually around 35 to 45 pounds, though this can vary depending on the mother's pre-pregnancy weight and overall health. A well-balanced diet rich in protein, healthy fats, and essential vitamins and minerals is crucial during a multiple pregnancy.

Women with multiple pregnancies are also monitored more closely for signs of preterm labor, as twins are more likely to be born prematurely than singletons. In some cases, medical interventions such as bed rest, medications to prevent preterm labor, or even hospitalization may be recommended to help prolong the pregnancy. However, every pregnancy is unique, and some women carrying twins or multiples reach full-term without significant complications.

Ultrasound technology plays a crucial role in managing multiple pregnancies. Regular ultrasounds allow healthcare providers to check for any growth discrepancies between the babies, monitor the amount of amniotic fluid, and assess the position of each baby in preparation for delivery. In cases where identical twins share a placenta, doctors will closely monitor for signs of twin-to-twin transfusion syndrome (TTTS), which occurs when blood flows unevenly between the twins and can lead to complications if left untreated. In such cases, early detection and intervention can improve outcomes, with treatments such as laser surgery to correct the blood flow imbalance.

Another important consideration in twin pregnancies is the mode of delivery. While many women with twins are able to have a vaginal delivery, others may require a cesarean section, particularly if one or both babies are in a breech position or if other complications arise. The decision about whether to deliver vaginally or via C-section depends on various factors, including the position of the babies, the mother's health, and the progress of labor. In some cases, a combination of both delivery methods may occur—for example, if the first baby is delivered vaginally but the second baby requires a C-section due to distress or positioning issues.

Emotional and Psychological Considerations for Multiple Pregnancies

While the medical aspects of twin and multiple pregnancies are often the focus of concern, it's equally important to address the emotional and psychological impact of carrying and raising multiples. Many parents-to-be experience a range of emotions when they find out they are expecting twins or more—excitement, joy, anxiety, and even fear. The idea of having two or more babies at once can feel overwhelming, especially for first-time parents or those who had not anticipated the possibility of multiples.

The increased physical demands of a multiple pregnancy can take a toll on a woman's mental and emotional well-being. Fatigue, discomfort, and the potential for complications can cause significant stress, and it's not uncommon for women carrying twins to feel anxious about their ability to carry the babies to term or manage the demands of parenting multiples. Additionally, many parents of multiples worry about the financial and logistical challenges of raising more than one baby at a time, such as the need for additional childcare, housing, and supplies.

It's important for expectant parents of twins or multiples to build a strong support system, both emotionally and practically. Partners, family members, and friends can offer valuable help during pregnancy and after the babies are born. Joining a support group for parents of multiples can also be beneficial, as it provides a space to connect with others who are going through similar experiences and challenges. These groups can offer practical advice, emotional support, and a sense of community that is especially valuable during the early years of raising multiples.

Counseling or therapy may also be helpful for parents who are feeling overwhelmed by the demands of a multiple pregnancy. Mental health professionals who specialize in prenatal and postpartum care can provide coping strategies for managing stress and anxiety, and they can help parents navigate the emotional complexities of preparing for twins or more.

Conclusion: The Truth About Twins and Multiple Pregnancies

Twins and multiple pregnancies are often surrounded by myths that can create unnecessary anxiety or unrealistic expectations. By debunking these myths and understanding the science behind how multiple pregnancies occur, parents and society can approach the experience with greater knowledge and confidence.

The myth that twins only occur if they run in the family overlooks the many factors that can influence the likelihood of having multiples, including maternal age, fertility treatments, and random chance. Similarly, while twin pregnancies do come with increased risks, advances in prenatal care and medical technology have made it possible for most women carrying twins or multiples to have healthy pregnancies and deliveries.

Finally, understanding the emotional, psychological, and logistical challenges of raising multiples is just as important as addressing the medical aspects. By building a strong support system and seeking appropriate care, parents of twins and multiples can navigate the unique joys and challenges of their journey with confidence and resilience.

Twins and multiple pregnancies are a testament to the complexity and wonder of human reproduction. With the right information, support, and care, parents of multiples can embrace the experience with optimism and hope, knowing that while their journey may be different from those expecting singletons, it is no less rewarding.

Misleading Myths About Pregnancy Loss and Fertility

Pregnancy loss and fertility are topics that often carry a heavy emotional burden for individuals and couples trying to conceive. Along with the emotional weight, these issues are surrounded by numerous myths and misconceptions that can cause further distress, confusion, and guilt. Misleading beliefs about miscarriage, fertility, and assisted reproductive technologies, such as in vitro fertilization (IVF), often exacerbate the difficulties that many people already face on their fertility journey. This chapter addresses some of the most common myths regarding pregnancy loss and fertility, and provides evidence-based information to separate fact from fiction.

Myth 27: Miscarriages Are Always Caused by Something the Mother Did

One of the most damaging myths surrounding pregnancy loss is the belief that miscarriages are always caused by something the mother did or failed to do. This myth perpetuates the notion that mothers bear full responsibility for the outcome of their pregnancies, which can lead to intense guilt, shame, and self-blame for women who experience a miscarriage. The reality, however, is that the vast majority of miscarriages are not caused by anything the mother did, and many occur due to factors that are completely out of her control.

Miscarriages, which occur in approximately 10-20% of known pregnancies, are most commonly caused by chromosomal abnormalities in the embryo. These genetic abnormalities happen randomly during the process of fertilization and early development, often because the embryo has an incorrect number of chromosomes. When an embryo has too many or too few chromosomes, it typically cannot develop properly, resulting in a miscarriage. These chromosomal abnormalities are usually not inherited and are unlikely to recur in future pregnancies.

In addition to chromosomal abnormalities, other factors can contribute to miscarriage, such as problems with the uterus (e.g., uterine fibroids or structural abnormalities), hormonal imbalances (such as insufficient levels of progesterone), or certain medical conditions like uncontrolled diabetes or thyroid disorders. In some cases, infections or autoimmune disorders may also increase the risk of miscarriage, but these are relatively rare.

While lifestyle factors like smoking, excessive alcohol consumption, and drug use can increase the risk of miscarriage, most women who experience a miscarriage did nothing to cause it. Normal activities such as exercising, lifting moderate weights, having sex, or experiencing emotional stress do not typically lead to miscarriage. Unfortunately, the myth that mothers are always responsible for their pregnancy loss can cause them to unfairly scrutinize every action they took during pregnancy, even when those actions were entirely unrelated to the loss.

It is important to understand that miscarriage is a natural, though painful, part of the reproductive process. In many cases, miscarriage occurs because the body recognizes that the embryo is not viable and cannot develop into a healthy baby. This biological mechanism, though devastating for the parents, is often beyond anyone's control. By dispelling the myth that miscarriage is caused by something the mother did, we can help alleviate the unnecessary guilt and self-blame that many women experience after a pregnancy loss.

Support from healthcare providers, family, and friends is essential in helping women and their partners navigate the grief and emotional healing process following a miscarriage. Counseling and support groups can also provide valuable resources for processing the loss and preparing for future pregnancies. Most women who experience a miscarriage go on to have healthy pregnancies and babies in the future, and it is crucial to offer hope and reassurance during such a difficult time.

Myth 28: Infertility is Rare in Women Under 35

A common misconception is that infertility is a condition that only affects older women, particularly those over the age of 35. While it is true that fertility declines with age, the myth that infertility is rare in younger women is misleading and can create a false sense of security for those trying to conceive. In reality, infertility can affect women of all ages, including those under 35, and it is important to recognize that reproductive challenges are not limited to older women.

Infertility is typically defined as the inability to conceive after one year of regular, unprotected intercourse for women under 35, or after six months for women over 35. While the chances of infertility do increase with age—due to factors such as declining egg quality and quantity—approximately 10-15% of women of reproductive age experience infertility, and this includes younger women.

There are several reasons why younger women may experience infertility, many of which are unrelated to age. Conditions such as polycystic ovary syndrome (PCOS), endometriosis, and thyroid disorders can affect ovulation and make it difficult for women to conceive, even in their 20s and early 30s. PCOS, for example, is one of the most common causes of infertility in women of reproductive age, affecting approximately 6-12% of women worldwide. It is characterized by irregular menstrual cycles, an excess of male hormones (androgens), and the presence of multiple small cysts on the ovaries, all of which can disrupt normal ovulation.

Endometriosis, a condition in which tissue similar to the lining of the uterus grows outside the uterus, can also cause infertility by affecting the ovaries, fallopian tubes, and pelvic organs. Women with endometriosis often experience pain and heavy periods, but the condition can also impair fertility by creating inflammation or scar tissue that interferes with the fertilization process.

Additionally, lifestyle factors such as being underweight or overweight, smoking, excessive alcohol consumption, and exposure to environmental toxins can also contribute to infertility in women of all ages. In some cases, male factor infertility—such as low sperm count or motility—may be the underlying cause, emphasizing the need for both partners to undergo fertility evaluations if they are having difficulty conceiving.

For younger women who are struggling with infertility, early intervention and medical evaluation are key. While age-related infertility may not be a concern for women under 35, addressing underlying medical conditions, hormonal imbalances, or other factors that could be contributing to infertility is essential for increasing the chances of conception. Fertility treatments such as ovulation-stimulating medications, intrauterine insemination (IUI), or IVF may be recommended depending on the cause of infertility.

The myth that infertility is rare in younger women can lead to delays in seeking help, as many women assume that their fertility issues will resolve naturally over time. By understanding that infertility can affect women at any age, couples can seek the appropriate medical care and support earlier in their journey, increasing their chances of a successful pregnancy.

Myth 29: IVF Guarantees a Successful Pregnancy

In vitro fertilization (IVF) is one of the most well-known and widely used assisted reproductive technologies (ART) available today. It offers hope to couples who are struggling with infertility, and it has helped millions of people around the world achieve their dream of parenthood. However, a common myth about IVF is that it guarantees a successful pregnancy, leading many individuals and couples to believe that IVF is a foolproof solution to their fertility struggles. While IVF can be highly effective, it is not without its challenges, and success is not guaranteed for every patient.

The process of IVF involves stimulating the ovaries to produce multiple eggs, retrieving those eggs, fertilizing them with sperm in a laboratory, and then transferring one or more embryos back into the uterus. IVF is often used in cases where other fertility treatments have failed, or in situations where specific medical conditions—such as blocked fallopian tubes, male factor infertility, or unexplained infertility—make natural conception difficult or impossible.

While IVF offers hope to many, the success rates of IVF can vary significantly depending on a number of factors, including the woman's age, the cause of infertility, the quality of the embryos, and the specific fertility clinic or treatment protocol used. For women under 35, the success rate of IVF per cycle is typically around 40-50%. However, success rates decline with age, with women over 40 having a significantly lower chance of a successful pregnancy. By the age of 43, the success rate of IVF may drop to as low as 5-10% per cycle.

It is important to recognize that IVF is not a one-size-fits-all solution, and many patients require multiple cycles of IVF before achieving a successful pregnancy. Each cycle of IVF involves a financial, emotional, and physical commitment, as the process can be expensive, stressful, and physically demanding. Hormonal medications used to stimulate egg production can cause side effects such as bloating, mood swings, and discomfort, and the egg retrieval process itself is a minor surgical procedure.

In addition to the potential physical challenges, the emotional toll of undergoing IVF can be significant, particularly for those who have experienced previous pregnancy losses or failed fertility treatments. The anticipation of each IVF cycle, followed by the waiting period to find out whether the cycle was successful, can create a roller coaster of emotions for individuals and couples hoping to conceive.

It is also worth noting that while IVF can increase the chances of conception, it does not guarantee that the pregnancy will be free from complications. Miscarriage, ectopic pregnancy, and other pregnancy-related issues can still occur following IVF, and patients must be prepared for the possibility that their journey to parenthood may involve setbacks.

Despite these challenges, IVF remains one of the most effective fertility treatments available, and many people go on to have healthy pregnancies and babies through this method. However, it is crucial to approach IVF with realistic expectations and an understanding that success is not guaranteed. By working closely with a fertility specialist and discussing individual factors that may affect IVF success, patients can make informed decisions about their treatment options.

Fertility and Pregnancy Loss: Facts vs. Fiction

The myths surrounding fertility and pregnancy loss are deeply ingrained in society, often perpetuated by misinformation, cultural beliefs, and outdated medical understanding. These myths can cause significant emotional distress for individuals and couples facing fertility challenges, leading them to question their own actions, bodies, and worthiness as parents. It is essential to replace these myths with facts so that people can approach their fertility journey with accurate information, compassion for themselves, and a realistic understanding of the challenges they may face.

First, it is important to acknowledge that pregnancy loss and fertility challenges are common and often unrelated to any actions or failures on the part of the individuals involved. As discussed earlier, the majority of miscarriages are caused by chromosomal abnormalities, not something the mother did or failed to do. Fertility issues can affect people of all ages, genders, and backgrounds, and they are often the result of medical conditions or factors beyond one's control, such as genetic predispositions, environmental exposures, or underlying health conditions.

The first step toward dispelling the myths around pregnancy loss and fertility is recognizing that these challenges are not uncommon. According to the Centers for Disease Control and Prevention (CDC), approximately 10% of women in the U.S. between the ages of 15 and 44 experience difficulty getting pregnant or staying pregnant. Additionally, about 10-20% of known pregnancies end in miscarriage, with many more occurring so early that they go undetected. These statistics underscore the reality that fertility struggles and pregnancy loss are part of the reproductive journey for many individuals and couples.

Support and education are key to navigating these challenges in a healthy, informed manner. Medical professionals can provide essential guidance, helping to clarify misconceptions about fertility and pregnancy loss. Access to fertility specialists, genetic counselors, and reproductive endocrinologists can empower individuals to make informed decisions about their fertility treatment options, whether they are considering IVF, intrauterine insemination (IUI), or other interventions.

It is also important for people to have realistic expectations when it comes to fertility treatments. While options like IVF have revolutionized fertility care and made parenthood possible for millions of people worldwide, they are not a guarantee of success. IVF success rates vary depending on a variety of factors, including age, the underlying cause of infertility, and the quality of care. Even with the most advanced technology, achieving pregnancy through IVF may require multiple attempts and involve significant emotional, physical, and financial investments.

Another critical aspect of addressing these myths is the normalization of conversations around fertility struggles and pregnancy loss. Many people feel isolated or ashamed when faced with these challenges, fearing judgment or misunderstanding from friends, family, or even healthcare providers. This silence only perpetuates the stigma surrounding fertility issues, making it harder for people to seek help or find support when they need it most.

By fostering open, compassionate discussions about these topics, we can create a more supportive environment for those facing fertility challenges. Whether through online communities, support groups, or one-on-one conversations, sharing experiences can help individuals and couples feel less alone and more empowered to navigate their fertility journey. Moreover, normalizing these conversations can help dispel harmful myths and provide accurate information to people who may be relying on outdated or incorrect beliefs about fertility and pregnancy loss.

It is also important to recognize that the path to parenthood is different for everyone. For some, fertility treatments like IVF may eventually lead to a successful pregnancy. For others, the journey may involve alternative routes, such as adoption, surrogacy, or choosing to live without children. Each of these paths is valid, and there is no single "right" way to build a family. What matters most is that individuals and couples have access to the information, resources, and support they need to make informed, empowered choices about their reproductive health and family-building journey.

Finally, the emotional impact of fertility struggles and pregnancy loss cannot be overstated. The grief, frustration, and uncertainty that often accompany these experiences can be overwhelming, and it is important for people to prioritize their mental and emotional well-being throughout the process. Therapy, counseling, and support groups can offer valuable tools for coping with the emotional ups and downs of fertility treatments and pregnancy loss. Partners and family members can also play a crucial role in providing emotional support, helping to alleviate feelings of isolation or helplessness.

In conclusion, debunking the myths surrounding fertility and pregnancy loss is essential for fostering a more compassionate and informed approach to reproductive health. By understanding the true causes of miscarriage, acknowledging that infertility can affect women of all ages, and recognizing that no fertility treatment guarantees success, we can help individuals and couples make more informed decisions about their reproductive journeys. Ultimately, the goal is to provide support, accurate information, and empathy to those facing the challenges of fertility and pregnancy loss, empowering them to navigate their unique paths to parenthood with confidence and hope.

Pregnancy and Beauty

Pregnancy is often depicted as a time when women radiate beauty and vitality, with glowing skin, luxurious hair, and an overall sense of well-being. These idealized portrayals contribute to the perception that pregnancy transforms a woman's appearance in universally positive ways. However, as with many aspects of pregnancy, there are a host of beauty-related myths that can create unrealistic expectations or cause unnecessary worry when those idealized outcomes do not come to pass. The reality is that every woman's body responds differently to pregnancy, and the changes to skin, hair, and appearance are highly individual. Some women may indeed experience the much-touted pregnancy glow, while others may face challenges like acne, hair thinning, or stretch marks. In this chapter, we will explore some of the most common beauty myths surrounding pregnancy and separate fact from fiction to provide a clearer understanding of what to expect when it comes to changes in appearance during pregnancy.

Myth 30: Your Hair and Skin Will Glow Throughout Pregnancy

One of the most pervasive myths about pregnancy is the idea that a woman's hair and skin will "glow" throughout the entire nine months. The concept of the "pregnancy glow" has become deeply ingrained in popular culture, with many expecting that all pregnant women will exude a healthy, radiant appearance. While some women do experience a noticeable improvement in their skin and hair during pregnancy, this is not the case for everyone, and the reasons behind these changes are more complex than they might seem.

The so-called pregnancy glow is often attributed to hormonal changes that occur during pregnancy. Increased levels of estrogen and progesterone stimulate blood flow to the skin, which can give the complexion a brighter, more radiant appearance. Additionally, the body produces more oil (sebum) during pregnancy, which can create a natural sheen or "glow" on the skin. However, this increase in oil production can also have the opposite effect for some women, leading to acne or other skin issues, particularly if they are prone to oily skin or breakouts.

Hormonal fluctuations during pregnancy can also impact hair. Many women experience fuller, thicker hair during pregnancy due to a prolonged growth phase in the hair cycle. Normally, hair goes through a cycle of growth, rest, and shedding, but during pregnancy, the increased levels of estrogen slow down the shedding phase, leading to the appearance of thicker, more voluminous hair. This effect is usually most noticeable in the second and third trimesters.

However, not all women experience this hair boost. Some may notice changes in hair texture or even hair thinning during pregnancy, particularly if they have underlying conditions such as thyroid disorders or nutritional deficiencies that can affect hair health. In fact, hair growth can be highly variable during pregnancy, and for some women, the supposed "glow" may be accompanied by issues like dull or brittle hair.

Moreover, the "glow" associated with pregnancy is often temporary. After giving birth, many women experience postpartum hair shedding (telogen effluvium), which can result in significant hair loss as the hair follicles return to their normal growth cycle. This is a natural part of the postpartum process, but it can be distressing for women who became accustomed to the thicker hair they enjoyed during pregnancy. The hair typically returns to its pre-pregnancy state within six to twelve months after childbirth.

The myth of the pregnancy glow can lead to disappointment or concern for women whose skin and hair do not conform to these idealized expectations. It's important to remember that every woman's body responds differently to pregnancy hormones, and not everyone will experience the same changes. Some women may see improvements in their skin and hair, while others may face new challenges, such as acne, hyper-pigmentation (often referred to as the "mask of pregnancy" or melasma), or changes in hair texture. These changes are all part of the natural variability of pregnancy, and none are an indication of a "better" or "worse" pregnancy experience.

Myth 31: Stretch Marks Are Unavoidable

Another common beauty myth is the belief that stretch marks are an unavoidable part of pregnancy and that there is little a woman can do to prevent them. Stretch marks, known medically as striae gravidarum, are a type of scarring that occurs when the skin stretches rapidly, such as during pregnancy. These marks often appear on the abdomen, breasts, thighs, or hips as the skin stretches to accommodate the growing baby and increased body size.

While it is true that many women develop stretch marks during pregnancy—studies suggest that between 50% and 90% of pregnant women experience them—it is not inevitable for everyone, and their development depends on a variety of factors. Genetics plays a significant role in whether a woman will develop stretch marks. If a woman's mother or other female relatives had stretch marks during pregnancy, she may be more likely to develop them as well. Additionally, the degree of weight gain and how quickly the skin stretches can influence the likelihood of developing stretch marks.

The skin's elasticity is another factor that determines whether stretch marks will form. Women with more elastic skin are less likely to develop stretch marks, whereas those with less elastic skin may be more prone to them. Skin elasticity is largely influenced by genetics, but factors such as hydration, nutrition, and overall skin health can also play a role.

There is a widespread belief that applying creams, oils, or lotions during pregnancy can prevent or minimize stretch marks. While moisturizing the skin can help keep it supple and hydrated, research on the effectiveness of topical treatments in preventing stretch marks is mixed. Some studies suggest that products containing ingredients like cocoa butter, shea butter, vitamin E, or hyaluronic acid may help reduce the appearance of stretch marks, but no treatment has been proven to completely prevent them. In many cases, the development of stretch marks is more closely related to genetics and the rate of skin stretching than to the use of any particular product.

It is also important to note that stretch marks, while they may initially appear red, purple, or dark brown, typically fade over time. As the skin heals, the marks become lighter in color and less noticeable, although they may not disappear completely. For women who are concerned about the appearance of stretch marks postpartum, there are options such as laser treatments or microneedling that can help improve the texture and appearance of the skin.

Ultimately, while stretch marks are a common part of pregnancy for many women, they are not unavoidable, and their development depends on a combination of genetic and environmental factors. For those who do develop stretch marks, it's important to recognize that these marks are a natural part of the body's transformation during pregnancy, and they should not be seen as a flaw or imperfection. Many women come to embrace their stretch marks as a symbol of the strength and resilience of their bodies during pregnancy and childbirth.

Fact-Checking Beauty Myths During Pregnancy

In addition to myths about glowing skin and stretch marks, there are many other beauty-related myths that circulate during pregnancy. These myths often contribute to unrealistic expectations about how a woman's body should look or behave during this time, and they can create unnecessary anxiety or pressure to conform to idealized beauty standards. Here, we will explore and fact-check some of the most common beauty myths during pregnancy.

Myth: Pregnancy always improves your nails.

It is true that some women notice stronger, faster-growing nails during pregnancy due to hormonal changes and increased blood circulation. However, this is not the case for everyone. Some women may experience brittle or weak nails, particularly if they have underlying nutritional deficiencies or if their body is directing most of its resources toward supporting the growing baby. Nails, like hair and skin, respond differently to pregnancy hormones depending on the individual.

Myth: Pregnant women should avoid all skincare products.

While it's true that certain skincare ingredients, such as retinoids and salicylic acid, should be avoided during pregnancy due to potential risks to the developing baby, many skincare products are safe to use. Ingredients like hyaluronic acid, glycerin, and gentle cleansers can help keep the skin hydrated and healthy during pregnancy without posing any risk to the baby. Sunscreen, in particular, is essential during pregnancy, as hormonal changes can make the skin more sensitive to the sun and more prone to developing melasma or other pigmentation issues.

It's always best to consult with a healthcare provider or dermatologist to ensure that any skincare products being used during pregnancy are safe. Additionally, many pregnancy-safe products are specifically formulated to address common skin concerns during pregnancy, such as dryness, stretch marks, or acne.

Myth: You can't dye your hair while pregnant.

The concern over hair dye during pregnancy stems from the fear that the chemicals in hair dye could be absorbed through the scalp and harm the developing baby. However, research on the use of hair dye during pregnancy has not shown any definitive evidence of harm. Most healthcare providers agree that it is safe to dye your hair during pregnancy, especially after the first trimester, when the baby's major organs have developed. If a woman is concerned about exposure to chemicals, she may opt for highlights (which don't touch the scalp), natural or ammonia-free dyes, or waiting until after the first trimester.

Myth: Pregnant women can't wear makeup.

Makeup is generally safe to use during pregnancy, but as with skincare products, it's a good idea to be mindful of the ingredients. Many pregnant women prefer to use makeup products that are free of harsh chemicals, parabens, or synthetic fragrances. Mineral-based makeup products, which tend to be gentler on the skin, are a popular choice for women who want to avoid potential irritants during pregnancy. Ultimately, wearing makeup during pregnancy is a personal choice, and there is no medical reason to avoid it as long as the products are safe.

Myth: Pregnancy always causes your hair to grow faster.

As mentioned earlier, hormonal changes during pregnancy can lead to thicker, fuller hair for some women, but this is not a universal experience. In some cases, women may experience hair thinning or changes in hair texture during pregnancy due to nutritional deficiencies, stress, or underlying medical conditions, such as thyroid imbalances. While many women do enjoy a period of more abundant hair growth during pregnancy, it is important to understand that hair responds differently to pregnancy hormones depending on the individual, and not every woman will experience thicker, faster-growing hair.

Additionally, any hair growth boost that occurs during pregnancy is temporary. After giving birth, many women experience a phase of increased hair shedding, known as telogen effluvium. This is because the high levels of estrogen that prolonged the hair's growth phase during pregnancy drop rapidly after delivery, causing more hairs to enter the resting phase and eventually fall out. This postpartum hair loss typically peaks around three to six months after giving birth and is a normal part of the body's adjustment back to its pre-pregnancy state. The hair usually returns to its normal growth cycle within a year after childbirth.

Fact-Checking Beauty Myths During Pregnancy: Summary

The idea that pregnancy always enhances a woman's physical appearance with glowing skin, thicker hair, and strong nails is a myth that fails to account for the wide range of experiences women have during pregnancy. While some women do experience positive changes to their skin and hair, others may face challenges such as acne, dry skin, hair thinning, or stretch marks. These changes are all part of the natural variability of pregnancy, driven by hormonal fluctuations, genetics, and individual health factors.

It's important to approach these myths with a balanced perspective, recognizing that pregnancy affects every woman differently. The key is to focus on maintaining overall health and well-being, rather than striving to meet unrealistic beauty standards or expectations. Regular self-care, a healthy diet, proper hydration, and adequate rest can all contribute to a sense of well-being during pregnancy, but they do not guarantee the elimination of skin or hair challenges.

Women should feel empowered to care for their skin, hair, and nails in ways that make them feel comfortable and confident during pregnancy, whether that means using pregnancy-safe beauty products, seeking professional skincare advice, or simply embracing the natural changes their bodies are going through. Ultimately, pregnancy is a time of transformation, and the body's changes—both internal and external—are a reflection of the incredible process of bringing new life into the world.

Embracing Changes in Appearance During Pregnancy

It's important to remember that the physical changes experienced during pregnancy are a natural part of the process and reflect the body's remarkable ability to adapt to the demands of growing and nourishing a baby. While societal expectations and beauty myths may create pressure to "look a certain way" during pregnancy, it's essential for women to prioritize their health and emotional well-being above meeting external standards of beauty.

For some women, pregnancy may indeed come with benefits such as glowing skin, strong nails, and thicker hair, but for others, the experience may involve challenges like acne, hyper-pigmentation, or hair loss. Regardless of how the body responds, these changes are temporary, and they should not detract from the profound journey of pregnancy.

Women should feel free to embrace and celebrate their changing bodies, whether that means using beauty products that make them feel good, engaging in self-care routines, or simply accepting that their appearance may not match societal ideals during this time. By shifting the focus away from external appearance and toward physical and emotional health, women can cultivate a sense of empowerment and self-compassion throughout their pregnancy.

It's also important to have realistic expectations about postpartum changes. Many women feel pressure to "bounce back" to their pre-pregnancy appearance soon after giving birth, but the reality is that the body continues to undergo changes in the weeks and months following delivery. Postpartum hair shedding, stretch marks, and changes in skin texture are common, and it takes time for the body to recover fully. Rather than striving for an immediate return to pre-pregnancy form, women should focus on healing and supporting their bodies as they adjust to their new roles as mothers.

Conclusion: Beauty Myths in Perspective

Beauty myths surrounding pregnancy can create unrealistic expectations for women and contribute to unnecessary stress or disappointment. By debunking myths such as the idea that every woman will experience a pregnancy "glow" or that stretch marks are inevitable, we can help women approach their pregnancy journeys with a more realistic understanding of the changes their bodies may undergo.

Pregnancy is a time of transformation, both physically and emotionally, and each woman's experience is unique. Understanding that there is no single "right" way to look or feel during pregnancy allows women to embrace their individual journeys with confidence and self-compassion. By prioritizing health and well-being, and by making informed choices about skincare, haircare, and self-care routines, women can feel empowered to navigate the beauty myths of pregnancy without falling into the trap of unrealistic ideals.

In the end, pregnancy is about far more than physical appearance—it is a profound, life-changing experience that brings new life into the world. Whether or not a woman's skin glows or her hair thickens, the true beauty of pregnancy lies in the strength, resilience, and love that define this remarkable journey.

Myths About Baby Development

The development of a baby in the womb is an incredible process that has fascinated parents, scientists, and healthcare providers for centuries. From the moment of conception to the time of birth, a baby undergoes a remarkable transformation, growing from a single cell into a fully-formed human being. Along with this awe-inspiring development comes a host of myths and misconceptions about what a baby can and cannot do in utero. Many of these myths are rooted in outdated beliefs or incomplete scientific understanding, while others have been popularized by well-meaning but inaccurate advice. In this chapter, we will address some of the most common myths about baby development in the womb and explore what science really says about the capabilities and experiences of a developing fetus.

Myth 32: Babies Don't Feel Pain in the Womb

One of the most persistent myths surrounding fetal development is the belief that babies do not feel pain while they are in the womb. This misconception has significant implications, particularly in discussions about prenatal medical procedures or late-term abortions. While the issue of fetal pain is complex and often entangled in political and ethical debates, the scientific understanding of when and how a fetus develops the capacity to feel pain has evolved significantly in recent years.

The ability to feel pain is linked to the development of the nervous system, including the brain, spinal cord, and peripheral nerves. For a baby to perceive pain, these structures must be mature enough to transmit pain signals to the brain, and the brain must be capable of processing those signals. The development of these structures occurs gradually throughout pregnancy, and there is still some debate among scientists and medical professionals about the exact point at which a fetus can experience pain.

During the early stages of pregnancy, the nervous system is just beginning to form. By around 7 to 8 weeks of gestation, the first nerve cells start to appear, and by 12 weeks, the spinal cord and major nerve pathways are in place. However, the cerebral cortex—the part of the brain responsible for processing sensory information, including pain—does not begin to develop until around 20 weeks of gestation, and it is not fully functional until much later in pregnancy.

Based on current scientific evidence, most experts agree that the capacity for a fetus to experience pain likely begins around the third trimester, after 28 weeks of gestation. At this stage, the nervous system is sufficiently developed to transmit pain signals, and the brain is capable of processing those signals. Before this point, while a fetus may exhibit reflexive responses to stimuli, such as moving away from a touch or reacting to a sound, these responses are not necessarily indicative of the conscious experience of pain.

It is important to note that pain perception in a fetus is not the same as in a fully developed baby or adult. In utero, a baby is surrounded by amniotic fluid, which acts as a cushion, and the uterus provides a warm, protective environment. Additionally, some researchers suggest that the fetal brain may release natural pain-relieving chemicals, such as endorphins, to mitigate any discomfort the baby might experience during certain medical procedures or during birth itself.

While the question of fetal pain continues to be a topic of research and debate, it is clear that the ability to feel pain is linked to the development of the nervous system and brain. The myth that babies cannot feel pain in the womb is an oversimplification of a complex process, and it is essential to rely on scientific evidence when discussing issues related to fetal development and medical care during pregnancy.

Myth 33: Playing Music to Your Belly Makes Your Baby Smarter

Another widespread myth about baby development is the idea that playing music to your belly during pregnancy will make your baby smarter. This belief has been popularized by a variety of sources, from well-meaning parenting advice to products specifically marketed to expectant parents, such as prenatal headphones or "Mozart for Babies" albums. The idea that exposing a developing baby to music in utero could boost cognitive development, often referred to as the "Mozart Effect," is rooted in the assumption that early stimulation of the baby's brain will lead to increased intelligence or improved brain function after birth. However, the science behind this claim is far less definitive than popular culture would suggest.

The "Mozart Effect" originally gained attention in the 1990s after a study suggested that listening to Mozart's music could temporarily improve spatial reasoning abilities in college students. This finding was widely misinterpreted to suggest that exposure to classical music could increase intelligence, and the idea was quickly extended to the prenatal environment. Soon, products and recommendations emerged encouraging parents to play classical music to their unborn babies in the hopes of boosting their future intelligence.

However, subsequent research has not supported the idea that playing music to a baby in the womb has any measurable impact on intelligence or cognitive development. While it is true that babies can begin to hear sounds from the outside world as early as 18 to 20 weeks of gestation, and that by 24 weeks, they can respond to external sounds, there is no evidence to suggest that exposure to music in utero has any long-term While the science of fetal development offers an incredible glimpse into the intricacies of how a baby grows and matures in the womb, it's important to approach this knowledge with a sense of balance and realism. The myths surrounding baby development can sometimes lead to unnecessary stress for expectant parents, who may feel pressure to "do everything right" to ensure their baby is developing optimally. In reality, much of what happens in utero is guided by the body's natural processes, and while maternal health and environment are important, no single action is guaranteed to enhance or hinder a baby's development in dramatic ways.

One of the most important things expectant parents can do is to focus on maintaining their own well-being, as this directly contributes to a healthy pregnancy. This means attending regular prenatal checkups, following medical advice, eating a balanced and nutritious diet, staying active with pregnancy-safe exercises, and managing stress as effectively as possible. These actions can create a supportive environment for the baby's growth while also helping the mother feel more comfortable and confident throughout her pregnancy.

In addition to focusing on health, it's important to acknowledge that much of fetal development is beyond direct control. Genetic factors play a significant role in how a baby grows, as do random events during cell division and early development. This means that while lifestyle choices can influence certain aspects of pregnancy, many aspects of fetal development are simply a matter of biology and timing.

Nurturing a Connection with Your Baby

While debunking myths about fetal development is important, this doesn't mean that parents should avoid engaging with their baby in utero. Many expectant parents find great joy and emotional connection in talking to their baby, playing music, or gently massaging their belly. These activities can foster a sense of closeness and anticipation as the baby grows, even if they don't necessarily result in measurable changes in the baby's intelligence or behavior.

For example, talking or singing to your baby while they are in the womb can be a meaningful way to establish an emotional connection before birth. Studies have shown that babies can recognize their mother's voice and may even show a preference for it over other voices shortly after birth. This early recognition can play an important role in bonding during the postpartum period, as newborns are naturally comforted by familiar sounds from their prenatal environment.

Playing music to your baby can also be a soothing activity for both mother and child. While there is no evidence to suggest that listening to music will make a baby smarter, it can create a calming atmosphere for the mother, which in turn benefits the baby. Stress management is a key component of a healthy pregnancy, and relaxing activities like listening to music, meditating, or engaging in prenatal yoga can help reduce anxiety and promote emotional well-being.

The physical act of bonding with your baby during pregnancy—whether through touch, voice, or other forms of interaction—can also help prepare parents for the transition to parenthood. It creates opportunities to reflect on the upcoming changes, to visualize life with the baby, and to feel more connected to the pregnancy experience as a whole. These moments of connection are not only beneficial for emotional preparation but can also make the pregnancy journey feel more intimate and personal.

The Real Impact of the Prenatal Environment on Baby Development

While many myths about baby development in the womb focus on external influences like music or maternal emotions, the most significant factors affecting a baby's development are often related to the maternal environment. The health of the mother—both physical and emotional—plays a crucial role in shaping the prenatal environment and influencing the baby's growth.

Maternal nutrition is one of the most well-researched areas of prenatal care. A balanced diet that includes a variety of nutrients, vitamins, and minerals is essential for supporting both the mother's health and the baby's development. Certain nutrients, such as folic acid, iron, calcium, and omega-3 fatty acids, are particularly important for fetal growth. Folic acid, for example, is crucial for preventing neural tube defects, while omega-3s support brain and eye development. Proper hydration is also vital, as it helps maintain amniotic fluid levels and supports the body's increased blood volume during pregnancy.

In addition to nutrition, maternal stress levels can also impact the baby's development. High levels of chronic stress during pregnancy have been linked to preterm birth, low birth weight, and developmental issues later in life. While occasional stress is a normal part of life, managing stress effectively during pregnancy is important for both the mother's well-being and the baby's health. Techniques such as mindfulness meditation, prenatal yoga, and deep breathing exercises can help reduce stress and promote relaxation.

Another important consideration is exposure to environmental toxins. Pregnant women are advised to avoid exposure to certain chemicals and substances that could harm the developing fetus, such as tobacco smoke, alcohol, and certain medications. Additionally, avoiding exposure to environmental toxins like pesticides, heavy metals, and pollutants is recommended whenever possible. Reducing exposure to these harmful substances can minimize the risk of developmental problems and other pregnancy-related complications.

The Role of Genetics in Fetal Development

While the prenatal environment plays a significant role in shaping a baby's development, genetics are the foundation of fetal growth. From the moment of conception, a baby's genetic blueprint is determined by the combination of DNA from both parents. This genetic material contains the instructions for everything from eye color to the development of vital organs like the heart and brain.

Genetic factors influence many aspects of a baby's development, including physical traits, temperament, and even predispositions to certain health conditions. However, it's important to understand that genetics are not a rigid script—environmental factors can interact with genetics to influence outcomes. This concept, known as epigenetics, refers to how external factors like nutrition, stress, and toxins can affect how certain genes are expressed. For example, while a baby may inherit a genetic predisposition for a certain condition, environmental influences during pregnancy can either increase or decrease the likelihood that the condition will manifest.

Understanding the role of genetics in fetal development helps dispel myths about pregnancy interventions that promise to "boost" a baby's intelligence or alter their future abilities. While the prenatal environment is important, there are limits to what can be influenced by external factors. For example, no amount of playing classical music to the womb will alter a baby's genetic makeup or dramatically change their future intelligence. However, providing a supportive and healthy prenatal environment can help ensure that the baby's genetic potential is maximized, giving them the best possible start in life.

Preparing for Baby's Arrival: What Really Matters

As parents-to-be navigate the myths and realities of baby development, it's important to focus on what truly matters for a healthy pregnancy and a well-prepared arrival. Rather than becoming preoccupied with myths about intelligence-boosting activities or beauty standards during pregnancy, the focus should remain on creating a nurturing environment that prioritizes maternal and fetal health.

Prenatal care is a critical component of this preparation. Regular visits to a healthcare provider allow for monitoring of both the mother's and baby's health, ensuring that any potential issues are identified and addressed early. These appointments provide an opportunity to ask questions, discuss concerns, and receive evidence-based guidance on topics such as nutrition, exercise, and mental health.

It's also important for parents to take time to prepare emotionally and practically for the baby's arrival. This might involve attending prenatal classes, setting up the baby's nursery, or discussing birth plans with healthcare providers. Emotional preparation is just as important as physical preparation, and taking time to reflect on the changes that parenthood will bring can help ease the transition to life with a newborn.

Support networks are another key aspect of preparing for baby's arrival. Pregnancy is a time of both excitement and vulnerability, and having a strong support system—whether it's a partner, family members, or friends—can make a significant difference in a mother's experience. Surrounding oneself with positive influences, trusted healthcare providers, and supportive peers can create an environment where both mother and baby thrive.

Final Thoughts on Baby Development in Utero

The journey of baby development in the womb is a complex and remarkable process, shaped by genetics, the prenatal environment, and maternal health. While myths about pain perception, intelligence-boosting activities, and physical changes during pregnancy may persist, the reality is that a baby's development is influenced by a combination of biological and environmental factors that are unique to each pregnancy.

Expectant parents should focus on providing a healthy and supportive environment for their baby's growth while staying informed about what science really says about fetal development. By relying on evidence-based information and maintaining a balanced perspective, parents can approach pregnancy with confidence, knowing that they are doing everything they can to support their baby's well-being.

As exciting as it is to wonder about what a baby can see, hear, or feel in utero, the most important thing is ensuring a healthy pregnancy that gives both mother and baby the best chance for a safe and positive birth experience. Whether or not a baby "learns" from listening to music in the womb, what truly matters is the love, care, and connection that parents build with their child, both before and after birth.

COVID-19 and Pregnancy

The COVID-19 pandemic has brought significant uncertainty, particularly for vulnerable populations, including pregnant women. With the rise of the virus came an abundance of information and misinformation, leading to confusion about how COVID-19 affects pregnancy. As the pandemic unfolded, myths and fears spread rapidly, particularly surrounding the risks to pregnant women and their unborn babies. While early in the pandemic, there was limited knowledge about how the virus impacted pregnancy, the medical community has since gathered substantial data that dispels many of these fears. In this chapter, we will examine common myths about COVID-19 and pregnancy, explore what the latest research reveals, and provide clarity on how pregnant women can protect themselves and their babies during this ongoing global health crisis.

Myth 34: COVID-19 is Extremely Dangerous for Pregnant Women

One of the first myths to emerge during the pandemic was the belief that COVID-19 is extremely dangerous for all pregnant women, putting them at significantly higher risk of severe illness and complications. While it's true that pregnancy alters the immune system and can increase susceptibility to certain infections, the blanket statement that all pregnant women are at extreme risk from COVID-19 is misleading. The reality is more nuanced, and the level of risk depends on various factors, including the individual's health, vaccination status, and exposure to the virus.

Early in the pandemic, much of the fear surrounding COVID-19 and pregnancy stemmed from a lack of data and uncertainty about how the virus might affect pregnant women and their developing babies. The immune system undergoes changes during pregnancy to protect both the mother and the fetus, but this can sometimes make pregnant women more susceptible to viral infections. Past outbreaks of diseases like H1N1 influenza and SARS-CoV (another coronavirus) showed that pregnant women could experience more severe outcomes compared to the general population, leading to initial concerns that COVID-19 would have similar effects.

However, as more data became available, it became clear that while pregnant women are not universally at extreme risk, certain factors can increase their likelihood of experiencing severe illness if they contract COVID-19. According to the Centers for Disease Control and Prevention (CDC) and the World Health Organization (WHO), pregnant women who contract COVID-19 may be more likely to experience complications such as hospitalization, intensive care unit (ICU) admission, or the need for mechanical ventilation compared to non-pregnant women of the same age. This elevated risk is particularly true for those with underlying health conditions such as obesity, diabetes, heart disease, or respiratory issues, as well as those who are unvaccinated.

However, it is important to note that the majority of pregnant women who contract COVID-19 experience mild to moderate symptoms, and many recover without the need for hospitalization. The risk of severe outcomes is heightened for those with coexisting health conditions, and for these individuals, the virus can indeed pose a greater danger. Pregnant women with high-risk conditions should take extra precautions to avoid exposure to the virus and seek prompt medical care if they experience symptoms.

Additionally, studies have shown that COVID-19 infection during pregnancy can lead to increased risks of certain pregnancy-related complications, including preterm birth, preeclampsia, and stillbirth. However, these risks are not dramatically higher than those seen in the general population, and many women with COVID-19 have healthy pregnancies and deliver healthy babies.

Ultimately, while COVID-19 does present some risks for pregnant women—particularly those with underlying health conditions or severe cases of the virus—the idea that all pregnant women are at extreme risk is an exaggeration. Proper precautions, including vaccination, wearing masks, and practicing good hygiene, can help mitigate these risks, and most pregnant women who contract the virus recover without major complications.

Myth 35: Pregnant Women Shouldn't Get Vaccinated

One of the most pervasive and harmful myths to circulate during the pandemic is the belief that pregnant women should avoid getting vaccinated against COVID-19. Early on, this myth gained traction due to a lack of initial data on the safety of COVID-19 vaccines during pregnancy, as pregnant women were excluded from the first clinical trials. This absence of data led to uncertainty, and some healthcare providers were hesitant to recommend vaccination to pregnant patients until more information became available.

As a result, many pregnant women were left in a state of confusion, torn between the desire to protect themselves from the virus and fears about the potential risks of vaccination during pregnancy. Misinformation on social media and other platforms only compounded these fears, with false claims suggesting that the vaccine could harm the developing baby, lead to infertility, or cause miscarriage.

However, as more research has been conducted, the evidence overwhelmingly supports the safety and efficacy of COVID-19 vaccines for pregnant women. Multiple studies have shown that the mRNA vaccines (such as Pfizer-BioNTech and Moderna) are safe for use during pregnancy and do not increase the risk of miscarriage, preterm birth, or other pregnancy complications. In fact, getting vaccinated is one of the most effective ways for pregnant women to protect themselves and their babies from the potentially severe effects of COVID-19.

According to the CDC, vaccination during pregnancy is strongly recommended, as it not only protects the mother from severe illness but also provides passive immunity to the baby. Antibodies generated by the mother in response to the vaccine can cross the placenta and provide some level of protection to the baby after birth. This is particularly important because newborns and infants are not eligible for COVID-19 vaccination, so maternal antibodies can help shield them from the virus during the early months of life.

Moreover, research has shown that pregnant women who contract COVID-19 are at an increased risk of severe illness and pregnancy complications, especially if they are unvaccinated. Vaccination significantly reduces the likelihood of hospitalization, severe outcomes, and death from COVID-19, making it a crucial tool in safeguarding maternal and fetal health.

It's also important to dispel the myth that COVID-19 vaccines can cause infertility. This false claim has been thoroughly debunked by experts in reproductive health. The mRNA vaccines do not interact with the DNA in cells, and there is no scientific evidence to suggest that they affect fertility in women or men. Studies have also shown that vaccinated women do not experience higher rates of miscarriage or infertility compared to unvaccinated women.

For pregnant women who are concerned about the vaccine, it is essential to have open, honest discussions with healthcare providers. Medical professionals can provide the latest research and personalized recommendations based on individual health factors, helping women make informed decisions about vaccination.

What We Now Know About COVID-19 and Pregnancy

As the pandemic has progressed, our understanding of how COVID-19 affects pregnant women and their babies has deepened significantly. While there are still some unanswered questions, the available data provide a clearer picture of the risks and protective measures that are essential during pregnancy.

One of the most important findings is that pregnant women are at higher risk for severe illness from COVID-19 compared to non-pregnant women, particularly if they have underlying health conditions. This increased risk includes complications such as pneumonia, acute respiratory distress syndrome (ARDS), and the need for intensive care. In severe cases, COVID-19 can also increase the risk of maternal mortality.

At the same time, the risk to the fetus is a key area of concern. Studies have shown that pregnant women with COVID-19 are more likely to experience pregnancy complications such as preterm birth, which can lead to health challenges for the newborn. There is also some evidence to suggest that maternal infection may increase the risk of stillbirth, although this remains relatively rare. However, these risks are more pronounced in cases where the mother experiences severe illness, underscoring the importance of vaccination and preventive measures.

Vertical transmission of the virus (from mother to baby) during pregnancy appears to be relatively uncommon. While there have been some cases where newborns tested positive for COVID-19 shortly after birth, it is unclear whether the transmission occurred in utero or after delivery. Most newborns born to mothers with COVID-19 do not test positive for the virus, and the majority of babies who do contract COVID-19 experience mild or asymptomatic cases. However, newborns can still be vulnerable to severe illness, particularly if they have underlying health conditions or are born prematurely.

The pandemic has also brought increased attention to the importance of mental health during pregnancy. Pregnant women have faced unique stressors during the COVID-19 crisis, including concerns about their health, isolation due to social distancing measures, and uncertainty about the safety of prenatal care and delivery. This heightened stress can have both physical and emotional effects on the mother and baby, making mental health support an essential part of prenatal care during the pandemic. Many healthcare providers now offer virtual consultations or telehealth services to help pregnant women navigate the challenges of pregnancy during COVID-19 while minimizing the risk of exposure to the virus.

In terms of treatment, pregnant women with COVID-19 are eligible for the same antiviral therapies and supportive care as non-pregnant patients, including monoclonal antibody treatments. These treatments can help reduce the severity of symptoms and prevent the progression of the disease, especially when administered early in the course of infection.

In conclusion, the fear and confusion surrounding COVID-19 and pregnancy have given rise to numerous myths, many of which have been debunked by emerging scientific research. While pregnant women are at a higher risk of severe illness from COVID-19, especially if they are unvaccinated or have underlying health conditions, the majority of pregnancies progress without major complications. Vaccination remains the most effective tool in protecting both mothers and their babies from the virus, and it offers the added benefit of passing protective antibodies to the newborn.

As we continue to learn more about COVID-19, it is clear that a balanced approach—focused on science, preventive care, and emotional support—is key to ensuring healthy pregnancies during the pandemic. By separating fact from fear, expectant mothers can make informed decisions about how to protect themselves and their babies while navigating the challenges of pregnancy in a global health crisis.

Busting Modern- Pregnancy Trends

Pregnancy is a time of excitement and anticipation, but it can also be a period filled with uncertainty, especially for first-time mothers. The wealth of information available, particularly online, has made it easier than ever to access advice on pregnancy and childbirth. However, the rise of social media, blogs, and influencers has also led to the proliferation of pregnancy trends and wellness products that are often more rooted in marketing than in science. While some modern pregnancy trends are harmless and might even provide comfort or entertainment, others can be misleading, unnecessary, or even potentially harmful. In this chapter, we will explore some of the most popular trends and products marketed to pregnant women, and debunk the myths surrounding them. From viral social media challenges to must-have gadgets, we will separate fact from fiction to help expectant mothers make informed choices during this special time.

Myth 36: Social Media Pregnancy Trends You Should Ignore

Social media platforms such as Instagram, TikTok, and YouTube are overflowing with pregnancy-related content, from glowing influencers sharing their daily pregnancy routines to viral challenges that claim to help with pregnancy symptoms or predict the baby's gender. While many of these trends are shared with good intentions, the reality is that much of the information circulating on social media is based on anecdotal evidence or pseudoscience, and it's crucial to approach these trends with a healthy dose of skepticism.

One of the most common social media trends is the use of DIY gender prediction tests. These viral videos often show expectant parents performing various at-home experiments, such as mixing baking soda with urine or observing the color of certain foods after exposure to heat, to determine the baby's sex. Despite their popularity, there is no scientific basis for these methods, and they are little more than fun activities. The only reliable ways to determine a baby's gender before birth are through medical procedures such as ultrasound (typically performed around 18-20 weeks) or genetic testing.

Another widespread trend involves influencers promoting various "natural" methods to induce labor at home, such as eating certain foods, engaging in specific exercises, or even using herbal supplements. While many of these methods are harmless, some can pose risks to both the mother and the baby. For example, while there is anecdotal evidence that eating dates in the weeks leading up to labor may help soften the cervix, other popular suggestions, like castor oil, can cause complications such as dehydration or severe cramping. It is essential for pregnant women to consult their healthcare providers before attempting any methods to induce labor, as the safety and effectiveness of these methods can vary greatly.

Social media also perpetuates myths about what a "perfect" pregnancy should look like. Influencers often share highly curated images of their pregnancies, complete with immaculate nurseries, trendy maternity outfits, and glowing skin. While there is nothing inherently wrong with sharing the joyful moments of pregnancy, these images can create unrealistic expectations and put pressure on women to conform to idealized standards of beauty and wellness. In reality, pregnancy is a deeply personal and individual experience, and no two pregnancies are the same. Comparing oneself to influencers or celebrities can lead to unnecessary stress, particularly when the realities of pregnancy—such as morning sickness, weight gain, and physical discomfort— don't match the picture-perfect images portrayed online.

It is also important to note that many influencers promoting pregnancy products or wellness trends are often compensated by brands, which can introduce bias into the advice they give. Pregnant women should be cautious of claims made by influencers or social media personalities, especially when these claims are not backed by scientific evidence. Instead, they should seek information from reliable sources, such as healthcare providers or reputable medical organizations.

In short, while social media can provide a sense of community and support for pregnant women, it is essential to approach viral trends and advice with caution. What works for one person may not work for another, and it's always best to rely on evidence-based information when making decisions about pregnancy and childbirth.

Myth 37: Belly Bands and Other Must-Have Gadgets: Do They Work?

Pregnancy is often accompanied by physical discomfort, especially as the baby grows and the body adapts to the demands of supporting both mother and child. As a result, a wide variety of gadgets and products have been developed and marketed to help alleviate common pregnancy-related discomforts. One of the most popular products in this category is the belly band, which is designed to provide support to the lower back and abdomen during pregnancy. But do these gadgets really work, and are they necessary?

Belly bands, also known as maternity support belts, are elastic bands that wrap around the lower abdomen to offer support to the back and pelvis. They are often marketed as a solution for relieving pregnancy-related back pain, pelvic pain, and discomfort caused by the weight of the growing belly. While some women do find relief from using belly bands, it is important to understand that they are not a one-size-fits-all solution, and their effectiveness can vary depending on the individual.

For some women, especially those with conditions like pelvic girdle pain (PGP) or symphysis pubis dysfunction (SPD), belly bands can provide temporary relief by redistributing the weight of the belly and reducing strain on the lower back and pelvis. However, wearing a belly band is not a substitute for addressing the underlying causes of pain, such as weak abdominal muscles, poor posture, or pelvic misalignment. Women experiencing significant pain during pregnancy should consult a healthcare provider or a physical therapist, who can recommend exercises and stretches to strengthen the core and pelvic muscles and improve posture. In some cases, pelvic floor physical therapy may be recommended to help alleviate discomfort.

It's also important to use belly bands correctly. Wearing a support belt for too long or too tightly can cause discomfort and may lead to muscle weakness if the body becomes too reliant on external support. The key is to use belly bands as a supplemental tool for short periods rather than as a long-term solution. Additionally, it is essential to listen to your body—if wearing a belly band causes more discomfort, it may not be the right product for you.

Aside from belly bands, the pregnancy market is flooded with other "must-have" gadgets, ranging from prenatal massagers and posture correctors to specialized pillows and even pregnancy monitoring devices that claim to track the baby's movements or heart rate. While some of these products can provide comfort and peace of mind, others are unnecessary and may not offer any real benefit beyond what traditional methods can achieve.

For example, pregnancy pillows are widely popular, particularly U-shaped or C-shaped pillows that are designed to support the body while sleeping. These pillows can be helpful for women who have difficulty finding a comfortable sleeping position as their pregnancy progresses. They provide support for the back, hips, and belly and can help alleviate pressure on the joints. However, a regular body pillow or strategically placed standard pillows can often provide similar support, and there is no need to spend a lot of money on a specialized pregnancy pillow unless it provides significant comfort.

On the other hand, devices that claim to monitor the baby's movements or heart rate at home should be approached with caution. These gadgets, often marketed as Doppler or fetal heartbeat monitors, are not always reliable, and using them without proper medical training can lead to unnecessary anxiety or false reassurance. If a woman is concerned about her baby's movements or heartbeat, it is always best to contact a healthcare provider, who can conduct a proper assessment and provide professional guidance.

Ultimately, while some pregnancy gadgets can provide comfort and support, it's important to remember that many are not essential. Pregnant women should focus on maintaining a healthy lifestyle, staying active, and seeking professional advice for any pain or discomfort. Gadgets like belly bands or pregnancy pillows can be helpful for some, but they should not be seen as a replacement for proper medical care or physical therapy when needed.

Separating Fact from Fiction in Pregnancy Wellness Products

The pregnancy wellness industry has exploded in recent years, with a vast array of products claiming to support maternal health, ease pregnancy symptoms, or even enhance the baby's development. From supplements and teas to creams and lotions, many of these products are marketed as essential components of a healthy pregnancy. However, it's important to critically evaluate the claims made by these products and understand what science supports—and what it does not.

One of the most commonly marketed categories of pregnancy wellness products is stretch mark prevention creams and oils. These products often promise to prevent or reduce the appearance of stretch marks, a common concern for pregnant women as their bodies undergo rapid changes in size and shape. However, as discussed in an earlier chapter, stretch marks are largely influenced by genetics and the elasticity of the skin. While moisturizing the skin can help keep it hydrated and improve its overall appearance, there is little scientific evidence to suggest that any particular cream or oil can completely prevent stretch marks. Ingredients like cocoa butter, shea butter, and vitamin E are often touted as miracle ingredients for preventing stretch marks, but their effectiveness is largely anecdotal.

Similarly, prenatal vitamins are an essential part of a healthy pregnancy, but the market is flooded with supplements that go beyond the basic recommendations. While prenatal vitamins containing folic acid, iron, calcium, and DHA are recommended by healthcare providers to support fetal development, many brands offer additional ingredients that claim to boost energy, improve digestion, or enhance the baby's brain development. While these additional ingredients are often harmless, they may not provide any real benefit beyond a well-balanced diet and standard prenatal care. It's always best to consult with a healthcare provider before adding any new supplements to your routine, as some ingredients could interfere with medications or cause unwanted side effects.

Another area of concern is herbal teas and supplements marketed as "natural" remedies for pregnancy symptoms such as nausea, insomnia, or anxiety. While some herbal remedies can be safe and effective when used correctly, others may pose risks to both the mother and the baby. For example, certain herbs like raspberry leaf and nettle are often marketed as pregnancy-safe, but they should be used with caution and only under the guidance of a healthcare provider. Some herbs can have strong effects on the uterus or blood pressure, making them potentially dangerous during pregnancy, particularly if taken in large quantities or without proper medical supervision. For example, herbs such as blue cohosh and pennyroyal, which are sometimes marketed for labor induction, have been linked to serious complications, including uterine contractions and miscarriage. It's important for pregnant women to be cautious about using herbal supplements and to consult with a healthcare provider before trying any new herbal remedies.

Another wellness trend that has gained popularity in recent years is the use of essential oils during pregnancy. While essential oils like lavender, peppermint, and eucalyptus are often promoted for their relaxing and therapeutic properties, it's crucial to remember that not all essential oils are safe for use during pregnancy. Certain oils, such as rosemary, sage, and clary sage, can stimulate uterine contractions and should be avoided, particularly in the early stages of pregnancy. Additionally, essential oils should always be diluted properly before use and never ingested without medical guidance.

While essential oils can be helpful for managing certain pregnancy symptoms—such as nausea or headaches—when used safely and in moderation, pregnant women should be aware that "natural" does not always mean safe. Just like with any other wellness product, it's essential to research the ingredients and speak with a healthcare professional to ensure they are appropriate for pregnancy.

One of the most pervasive myths in the pregnancy wellness space is the idea that certain products or lifestyle changes can significantly alter the course of a pregnancy or improve the baby's health and development. For example, some products claim to boost the baby's intelligence, improve physical health, or increase chances of a smooth delivery. While many of these claims are marketed with persuasive language, they often lack scientific backing. The most effective ways to support a healthy pregnancy remain consistent: a balanced diet rich in essential nutrients, regular prenatal care, moderate physical activity, and proper rest. No wellness product can substitute for these fundamental practices.

Finally, it's important to address the increasing commercialization of pregnancy wellness, particularly through social media platforms where influencers promote products under the guise of personal testimonials. Many of these influencers are compensated for promoting products, and their recommendations may not be based on medical advice or personal experience with the product. This creates an environment where misinformation can spread rapidly, and pregnant women may feel pressured to purchase products that are unnecessary or ineffective.

To navigate the overwhelming world of pregnancy wellness products, pregnant women should focus on evidence-based recommendations from trusted healthcare professionals. While some products may offer comfort or minor benefits, the key to a healthy pregnancy lies in making informed choices based on scientific research rather than marketing hype. It's also essential to remember that every pregnancy is different, and what works for one person may not be necessary or beneficial for another.

Conclusion: Busting Modern Pregnancy Trends

Modern pregnancy trends and wellness products have created a booming industry, but they have also introduced a fair amount of confusion and misinformation. From social media-driven trends to must-have gadgets and wellness supplements, the market is saturated with products that promise to improve pregnancy experiences in ways that are often unsupported by science. While some of these products may provide comfort or entertainment, many are unnecessary, and some can even pose risks if used incorrectly.

Pregnant women must navigate this landscape with a critical eye, seeking out reliable, evidence-based information to make informed choices for their health and well-being. Healthcare providers remain the most trusted source for guidance during pregnancy, and their advice should always be prioritized over anecdotal claims or social media trends.

By debunking myths about pregnancy wellness products and modern trends, we can help expectant mothers focus on what truly matters: a safe, healthy pregnancy supported by proper prenatal care, balanced nutrition, and self-care practices tailored to their individual needs.

Conclusion

Pregnancy is one of the most trans-formative and deeply personal experiences a person can go through. It is a time filled with anticipation, joy, and a healthy dose of anxiety as expectant parents navigate the vast ocean of information available to them. In the modern world, where the internet, social media, and well-meaning friends and family are quick to offer advice, distinguishing between fact and fiction can be overwhelming. The truth is, much of the advice surrounding pregnancy is riddled with myths that, if not carefully examined, can lead to unnecessary stress, confusion, and even harmful choices. As we've discussed in earlier chapters, debunking these myths and fostering a culture of informed decision-making is essential for ensuring a healthier, happier pregnancy for both mother and baby.

The Importance of Informed Decision-Making in Pregnancy

One of the most critical aspects of pregnancy is the ability to make informed decisions. Informed decision-making means that expectant parents have access to accurate, evidence-based information that allows them to weigh the pros and cons of various choices. From understanding the importance of prenatal care and vaccinations to discerning which wellness products are safe, it is essential that all decisions be rooted in scientific fact, not fear or misinformation.

During pregnancy, many decisions must be made, and each of these decisions has an impact on both the mother and the baby. Whether it's deciding on a birth plan, choosing whether to receive certain vaccinations, or selecting appropriate nutrition and supplements, these choices should be made in collaboration with trusted healthcare providers. Having open, honest conversations with doctors and midwives ensures that expectant mothers receive guidance that is tailored to their unique circumstances and health needs.

Pregnancy, though a natural process, involves significant physiological changes, and every woman's body responds differently to these changes. Therefore, relying solely on anecdotal advice or following generalized trends can lead to misguided choices. For example, some women might be advised by friends to avoid exercise or to engage in certain behaviors based on outdated beliefs, but the reality is that each pregnancy is different. Medical advice should always be sought before making decisions about physical activity, diet, and other health-related issues during pregnancy.

One area where informed decision-making is especially crucial is in choosing whether to receive vaccinations, such as the COVID-19 vaccine. As discussed in previous chapters, the myth that vaccines are dangerous for pregnant women has been widely debunked by scientific research. However, lingering fears and misinformation can still influence a pregnant woman's decision. Informed decision-making allows individuals to weigh the risks and benefits based on facts, not myths, and to protect themselves and their babies from preventable diseases.

In addition to making decisions about medical care, expectant parents also need to navigate the world of wellness products and lifestyle trends. The booming pregnancy market is filled with products that claim to improve health, appearance, or comfort during pregnancy, but many of these products lack scientific backing. Whether it's belly bands, stretch mark creams, or herbal supplements, it's vital that pregnant women consult with healthcare professionals before using any new products. Not all "natural" products are safe, and some can interfere with medications or exacerbate underlying health conditions.

By focusing on informed decision-making, expectant parents can reduce anxiety and feel more empowered as they move through their pregnancy journey. When choices are made based on reliable information, mothers can be more confident in their ability to care for themselves and their growing babies, ultimately leading to better outcomes for both.

Embracing the Truth: How to Navigate Pregnancy with Confidence

Navigating pregnancy with confidence comes down to embracing the truth about what pregnancy entails, rather than succumbing to the myths and misinformation that often surround it. One of the first steps toward building this confidence is to accept that pregnancy is a highly individualized experience. No two pregnancies are exactly alike, and what works for one woman may not work for another. It is important for expectant mothers to listen to their own bodies and to trust the advice of healthcare professionals rather than attempting to conform to generalized expectations or social media trends.

Pregnancy is often portrayed in media and on social platforms as a time of glowing skin, thick hair, and boundless energy. While some women may experience these positive changes, many others face challenges such as morning sickness, fatigue, acne, or mood swings. These are normal parts of pregnancy, and it's essential to recognize that there is no "right" way to look or feel while pregnant. A pregnant woman's worth or health is not determined by how closely her experience aligns with idealized images. Instead, confidence comes from understanding that pregnancy is a unique journey with its own highs and lows, and that each woman's body is perfectly designed to go through this process in its own way.

Another critical aspect of navigating pregnancy with confidence is recognizing the importance of mental health. Pregnancy can bring about significant emotional and psychological changes, and it's normal for expectant mothers to experience feelings of anxiety, fear, or even depression. Unfortunately, there are still many myths surrounding mental health during pregnancy, such as the belief that pregnancy should be a time of constant happiness or that seeking help for mental health concerns is a sign of weakness. In reality, many women struggle with their mental health during pregnancy, and seeking support is one of the most empowering steps they can take.

Postpartum depression and anxiety are well-documented mental health conditions, but prenatal depression and anxiety are less commonly discussed. This can leave women feeling isolated or unsure of whether their feelings are valid. The truth is that mental health is just as important during pregnancy as physical health, and there is no shame in reaching out for help. Talking to a healthcare provider, joining a support group, or seeking therapy can provide pregnant women with the tools they need to cope with the emotional challenges of pregnancy.

By embracing the truth about the physical and emotional realities of pregnancy, expectant mothers can let go of the pressure to meet unrealistic standards and instead focus on their well-being. This allows them to build confidence in their ability to navigate pregnancy and childbirth, regardless of the challenges they may face along the way.

Final Thoughts on Debunking Myths for a Healthier, Happier Pregnancy

Pregnancy is a time of great change, both physically and emotionally, and it is easy to feel overwhelmed by the sheer volume of information—much of it conflicting—available to expectant parents. However, by debunking common myths and focusing on evidence-based practices, pregnant women can foster a healthier and happier pregnancy experience.

One of the key takeaways from debunking pregnancy myths is that it is essential to rely on science and medical expertise rather than on anecdotal stories or social media trends. For example, many women are told that they must "eat for two" during pregnancy, but this myth has been widely disprove. While it's important to increase caloric intake slightly to support the baby's growth, overeating can lead to unhealthy weight gain and complications such as gestational diabetes. Similarly, the idea that pregnant women should avoid all physical activity is outdated; in fact, regular exercise can have numerous benefits for both mother and baby, including reducing the risk of complications and improving mood and energy levels.

In the wellness market, products such as belly bands, essential oils, and herbal supplements are often marketed as "must-haves" for pregnancy. While some of these products can provide comfort, others offer little more than placebo effects, and some can even be dangerous if not used properly. By separating fact from fiction and focusing on proven methods of support—such as proper nutrition, prenatal care, and stress management—pregnant women can avoid unnecessary expenses and focus on what truly matters for their health.

The fear that often accompanies pregnancy can be alleviated through access to accurate, evidence-based information. For example, many women worry about the risks of receiving vaccines during pregnancy, but extensive research has shown that vaccines, such as the flu shot and COVID-19 vaccine, are safe and effective for both the mother and baby. In fact, they offer essential protection against diseases that can cause severe complications during pregnancy. By dispelling myths surrounding vaccines, healthcare providers can empower women to make choices that protect their health and the health of their unborn children.

In addition to the physical aspects of pregnancy, it's also important to debunk myths surrounding labor and delivery. Many women fear childbirth because of the pain and uncertainty associated with it, but modern medicine offers a variety of options for managing pain, including epidurals, medications, and natural techniques such as breathing exercises and labor positions. Birth plans can help women feel more in control of their experience, but it's also important to remain flexible, as labor is unpredictable. Debunking the myth that there is a "perfect" way to give birth helps women approach labor with a more open mindset and reduces feelings of failure if things don't go according to plan.

Finally, debunking myths about the postpartum period is equally important. Many women feel unprepared for the physical and emotional challenges they face after giving birth, in part because the focus of most pregnancy information is on the prenatal and birth phases. Myths such as the belief that breastfeeding is easy for all women or that a woman's body will quickly return to its pre-pregnancy state can set unrealistic expectations and contribute to postpartum anxiety or depression. By providing accurate information about the realities of postpartum recovery, including the possibility of breastfeeding challenges and the importance of mental health support, healthcare providers can help new mothers navigate this critical time with confidence.

In conclusion, pregnancy is a deeply personal journey, and while it can be filled with joy, it can also be marked by uncertainty, fear, and misinformation. By debunking common myths and promoting evidence-based practices, we can help expectant mothers make informed decisions that lead to healthier and happier pregnancies. Ultimately, the goal is to empower women to trust their bodies, their healthcare providers, and their own instincts as they navigate one of the most profound experiences of their lives. When pregnant women are equipped with the right information, they can approach pregnancy and childbirth with confidence, knowing they are making the best choices for themselves and their babies.

9 7 9 8 3 4 2 4 1 2 3 1 5